D0848035

EXISTENTIAL HYPNOTHERAPY

THE GUILFORD CLINICAL AND EXPERIMENTAL HYPNOSIS SERIES

EDITORS
MICHAEL J. DIAMOND AND HELEN M. PETTINATI

EXISTENTIAL HYPNOTHERAPY

Mark E. King, Ph.D.
Charles M. Citrenbaum, Ph.D.

THE GUILFORD PRESS
New York   London

© 1993 The Guilford Press
A Division of Guilford Publications, Inc.
72 Spring Street, New York, NY 10012

Printed in the United States of America

This book is printed on acid-free paper.

Last digit is print number: 9 8 7 6 5 4 3 2 1

Library of Congress Cataloging-in-Publication Data
King, Mark.
    Existential hypnotherapy / Mark E. King, Charles M. Citrenbaum.
        p.   cm. — (The Guilford clinical and experimental hypnosis series)
    Includes bibliographical references and index.
    ISBN 0-89862-344-8
    1. Hypnotism—Therapeutic use.   2. Existential psychotherapy.
    I. Citrenbaum, Charles.   II. Title.   III. Series.
    [DNLM: 1. Hypnosis—methods.   2. Existentialism.   WM 415 K53e 1993]
RC497.K46   1993
616.89'162—dc20
DNLM/DLC
for Library of Congress   93-25048
                                                                         CIP

To the old white oak,
the spiritual center of "home."

To Bonnie, the beautiful lady
who sits under the oak with me;
in this life a cross between an old
wise woman and a saloon singer.

To Michael and Kevin,
the explorers of the woods.

To Shana, Michele, and Jeffrey,
birds that now drift in the wind.
May you find fertile ground to land on.

To my parents,
with great appreciation for all their sacrifices.

M. E. K.

To my mother and my father.
To Jennifer, Anna, Katelyn, and Robert.

C. M. C.

Preface and Acknowledgments

In this text we are attempting to take the clinical hypnotherapy each of us has practiced for more than 20 years, taught in more than 300 workshops, and previously written about (Citrenbaum, King, & Cohen, 1985; King, Novik, & Citrenbaum, 1983) and organize it in terms of theoretical and philosophical principles. Existentialism is our guiding theory because it clearly articulates the world as we experience it.

You can be talked into some psychological theories because of their impressive internal logic and elaborate explanations and you can be impressed by other theories because extensive laboratory studies seem to validate different aspects of those theories. Psychoanalytic theory and learning theory are two such examples. But the only way you can become an existential thinker is if existential theory speaks to the world in which you already live. Often when we read the great existential writers we have an "Aha" experience. As soon as we read a certain passage we know intuitively that it is true (for us). In fact, the thought or insight seems so obvious to us that we wonder why the author bothered to write it down. Yet the thought is not exactly how we understood that aspect of the world previously, and herein lies the consciousness expansion that makes the theory valuable.

This book begins with several theoretical chapters that discuss the issues we think are important for psychotherapy in general and hypnotherapy in particular. Chapter 8 is also theoretical; it addresses the nature of diagnosis in general and the concept of addiction in particular. The other chapters focus on specific clinical issues and techniques as understood from an existential perspective. We understand hypnotherapy to be one type of psychotherapy; for those readers who do not use clinical hypnosis in their practice, in most cases the word *psychotherapy* can be substituted for *hypnotherapy* with little change in meaning.

This book is purposely short. Keeping it short took disciplined effort. We both believe that we are better clinicians than writers, probably because as therapists we learned the value of making the point and letting the patient struggle to understand it. The learning is in the struggle as well as in the point. When we write or teach we often fall into the trap Nietzsche described twice in *Human, All Too Human* (1984):

> Most thinkers write badly because they tell us not only their thoughts but also the thinking of the thoughts. (Aphorism 188)

> Even the most honest writer lets slip a word too many when he wants to round off a period. (Aphorism 191)

We owe thanks to many people. We wish to thank our wives, who are also our colleagues, Virginia Bonnie King and Carolyn Jennifer Golden; our good friends Richard Busch, Dr. Lew Morgan, and Dr. Jim Towe, all of whom read earlier drafts of our book and contributed to its improvement; Dr. William Cohen, from whom we learned much while sharing the stage with him at many hypnotherapy workshops; Colleen Scholl and Linda Helm for their help in preparing the manuscript; Sharon Panulla, our editor at The Guilford Press, and Susan Marples her associate; Dr. Michael J. Diamond, editor of The Guilford Clinical and Experimental Hypnosis Series; and Dr. James A. Hall, author of *Hypnosis: A Jungian Perspective*, who was kind enough to comment on the text. Finally, thanks to Natalie Goldberg and her beloved Taos Mountains for help with a writing block.

Contents

EXISTENTIAL HYPNOTHERAPY

Introduction to Existentialism

Interest in clinical hypnosis by mental health professionals reached an explosive level during the 1980s and continues unabated into the '90s. More books were written (as judged by selections of the major book services catering to professionals) and workshops taught on this topic than on any other mental health technique. (In the '90s perhaps only issues of sexual abuse and addiction have surpassed hypnosis.) Today a large number of clinicians have been trained via workshops or textbooks and use clinical hypnosis as part (unfortunately, some even use it as all) of their practice. Particularly popular is the work of Milton H. Erickson, who created the model of clinical hypnosis in which we were trained.

We have been particularly fortunate in our careers to have had the opportunity to travel across much of the country teaching hypnosis in professional settings. In our travels, we have noticed a serious shortcoming that affects the quality of treatment offered patients, a problem similar to the one that occurred in the 1970s when there was massive training in techniques such as gestalt therapy and transactional analysis; we are speaking of the lack of integration between the behavioral techniques in use and an integrated philosophy or psychological theory about the nature of psychotherapy. The most basic decisions of therapy—for example, when to use a particular technique, how to define mental health, how to set appropriate goals for a psychotherapy session, determining the requirements or limitations of one's professional behavior, determining what is to be expected (or demanded) of the patient—can only be understood and made within the context of a "larger picture" than knowledge of specific techniques. Too many of today's practitioners have theories of human development that are unarticulated, unexamined, unrefined, underdeveloped, and often unconscious to them (often derived from their own "early childhood hypnosis"— usually called socialization). This limits the therapist's ability to know which patients to work with, what techniques to use, when to use them, and when to terminate treatment. This text is an attempt to fill the gap between technique and therapy. We believe existential philosophy and psychology provides the best theoretical foundation for understanding the meaning of hypnotherapy, particularly when an Ericksonian approach to working with people is used.

Here, at the beginning, we must first distinguish between what we believe to be true for ourselves versus what we know to be true for all professionals who do psychotherapy and use clinical hypnosis. Regarding the latter, we believe that anyone who works with people in the mental health field and who has a well-conceived, integrated theory of personality and a unified philosophy will in the long run do better work than someone who lacks these things. It may well be that what theory one believes in does not really matter. We know of no empirical evidence good enough to cite here that would prove that only one theory is better than all the others. The significant difference exists between those possessed of deep integrated thinking versus those whose thinking is shallow and scattered. Many people from different theoretical backgrounds use clinical hypnosis as part of their work in the way that makes sense to them. For example, we can point to an excellent book in The Guilford Clinical and Experimental Hypnosis Series, *Hypnosis: A Jungian Perspective*, by James A. Hall (1989). Hall explains some basic principles of Jungian theory for those not familiar with it and then demonstrates how someone who adheres to the Jungian approach makes use of clinical hypnosis. We find his discussion of dreamwork most interesting. We hope others with different orientations will share the thinking behind their work.

What we believe to be true for ourselves (our existential reality, if you will) and what we believe makes the most sense for all those clinicians using an Ericksonian approach to hypnosis—but not limited to this group—is to use existential psychology, psychiatry, and philosophy to ground all clinical work, specifically the use of clinical hypnosis in a psychotherapy or medical setting. In the remainder of this text we will first discuss some of the basic existential theory that is relevant to the use of clinical hypnosis and then we will detail specific techniques that we believe to be consistent with this guiding philosophy.

EXISTENTIAL REALITY

Everyone familiar with clinical hypnosis has heard the term "Ericksonian hypnosis." Often people mistakenly believe that this type of hypnosis is merely a set of techniques for working with patients. For example, we have often heard that Erickson always made use of indirect communication techniques. People who believe this idea to be true have not spent much time watching old films and video tapes showing Erickson at work, for these films and videos reveal that he often gave direct commands to his patients. We often heard Erickson state that he hated the term "Ericksonian hypnosis"; indeed, he claimed that there was no such thing. However, we believe that Erickson was wrong in making this analysis of his own work because he did create an "approach" that was unique to him at the time, and we believe that it was very existential in its nature. Erickson was a genius when it came to discovering what made a patient "tick." He quickly understood how his patients experienced their lives, including their symptoms, and what was meaningful in *their* world. He literally made up an individual theory of personality for each person who walked into the office. One of the most frequently cited quotes from existential literature is Sartre's dictum from *Being and Nothingness* (1943): "Existence precedes essence." Erickson's approach was the ultimate actualization of this philosophy. He did not look at what would be considered a person's essence (such as ego structure or other preconceived personality theory traits), but instead looked at his or her existence, what life was like as he or she lived it. This understanding was the starting point of Erickson's intervention.

The principle involved here is so obvious and simple that we feel somewhat apologetic for making it; yet in our training of others, many of whom are experienced psychotherapists, we are amazed and disappointed to find that the principle is forgotten or misunderstood. In the mental health field the data clinicians work with is the patient's worldview, or what we call "existential reality"—it is not the "truth" in any metaphysical sense. The task of the psychotherapist is to work with a patient's reality and alter it when necessary in a way that is helpful to him or her. This idea is explained clearly and briefly by Paul Watzlawick (1984, 1985). He says that patients come to us with an understanding of the world that is in some way causing them pain; otherwise, they would not be in our offices. Our job is to help the patient exchange that painful worldview for a new one that is less painful. The new view is not necessarily any "truer" than the old one, but it should promote a healthier (and hopefully happier) life.

This attitude contrasts with the more traditional, often unarticulated, viewpoint in psychology according to which the therapist spends a lengthy period during the psychotherapy process searching for THE DIAGNOSIS and analyzing the historical truth of the patient's recall. Everyone is aware of clinicians who ignore what their patients tell them, such as "I smoke because it relaxes me on the job," and instead look for the "scientific truth"—in this case, nicotine dependency because it meets the criteria in DSM-III-R (American Psychiatric Association, 1987). This "truth" does not even begin to help change the patient's smoking behavior; indeed, the therapist's imposition of his or her "truth" on the patient is probably the major reason that most smoking cessation programs offered by professionals (including most using clinical hypnosis) have such a low success rate. How many clinicians have wasted hours of psychotherapy time trying to establish whether remembered sexual abuse actually occurred? This is a modern psychological chicken-and-egg question, a conundrum whose answer is really not necessary for successful treatment. What matters for therapy is the existential reality of your client—in this case, the experience of being an abuse victim.

Later, in Chapter 6, we will discuss ways to use the meaning a symptom has to the patient himself or herself to alter or eliminate that symptom. We believe that this approach is far more effective for the therapist than focusing on his or her own understanding of the disorder or symptom and trying to treat it from that perspective. Using the client's own reality as the basis of clinical work will also help the therapist to understand and ground highly effective trance work using images and metaphors that we will discuss in Chapter 7.

To do good existential psychotherapy and hypnosis one must develop what Shunryu Suzuki (1970) called "zen mind, beginner's mind." A master therapist, like a Zen master, has a beginner's mind, a mind empty of preconceptions and totally open to the experience or person in front of him or her. Hearing patients tell their stories, watching them as they do so, and feeling what it is like to be in the room with them enables the therapist to understand their realities, and to plan better interventions, but only if the therapist's mind is clear enough to perceive accurately.

HYPNOSIS

Let us begin with a question: What is hypnosis? The literature gives dozens of answers, most of which do not fit into an existential perspective. The word *hypnosis* itself is a metaphor based on the name of the Greek god of sleep, Hypnos. The word was coined in 1843 by Scottish physician James Braid to draw attention to what he saw as similarities between the behavior of sleepwalkers and what Mesmer was calling "animal magnetism." As a metaphor it is a helpful concept; understood as a descriptive term for a literal state of consciousness it is misleading. Trance, usually taken to mean the subject's experience during hypnosis, is often called an altered state of consciousness (Orne, 1959; Hilgard, 1965). This belief implies that there is one "state" or experience called regular or normal consciousness and that all deviations from this regular consciousness are altered states. To believe this, one needs to get away from a "beginner's mind" experience of the world and substitute a theory (an antiexistential one at that). Our daily reality has many forms of experience, each of which is a kind of consciousness, each of which has a thousand shades and faces. There is sleep (deep and light, with and without dreams), a barely alert early morning and late evening state, times of hyperattentiveness, and times when the mind seems to wander or not even be aware of itself. There is the subtle (and sometimes not-so-subtle) change that occurs in consciousness when everyday substances such as sugar and caffeine are ingested into or leave the body. There is the moment when we lose ourselves in the color of the fall leaves, or those moments of embarrassing self-awareness, and so on. Trance is yet another face of consciousness, but one given special meaning because of the relationship between the hypnotherapist who introduces trance to the patient and the experience called trance.

Trance is not sleep or a behavior resembling sleep, as suggested by some (for example, Goldenson, 1984). We ask patients to "alert" themselves at the end of a session, rather than to "wake up," a phrase many hypnotherapists inexplicably use. For most patients the experience of trance is different from the experience of sleep. Indeed, often patients may feel they have failed as subjects if sleep is the defining criterion used to measure "depth of trance." Moreover, the notion of being asleep, unaware and out of control of events, that many patients associate with trance, is not healthy. Indeed, the idea that they have no control over what happens while they are in trance is totally opposite to the reality of the therapeutic experience called trance.

One of the most frequently cited ideas about hypnosis is that all hypnosis is really some form of self-hypnosis (see Fromm & Kahn, 1990; Wright & Wright, 1987; Erickson, 1980, 1983). We started our training with Milton Erickson, and since he believed that hypnosis was really self-hypnosis, we believed and taught this idea for many years (Citrenbaum et al., 1985). When we decided "to stop being so smart," went back to "beginner's mind," and finally paid attention to our clients' experiences, we realized that trance could be understood *only* as part of the dialectical relationship between the psychotherapist who uses hypnosis and the patient who experiences the trance.

If hypnosis is anything (and it is difficult to say that a metaphor is any-*thing*), it is a cooperative process between subject and hypnotherapist. The patient somehow comes to believe that this process will be of benefit to him or her. Some believe in the benefits of hypnosis before they see us: that is why they chose a professional who uses this modality. Other patients need to be taught to believe in the value of hypnosis. In either case, we begin with a subject who engages in the process because he or she believes, totally or at least partially, that we, using this treatment, will help him or her. This is why they pay us, which is also part of the process. The relationship is a professional one. Hypnosis is a type of psychotherapy, but usually only part of a more complex and multifaceted treatment program. In the past, no matter how well we thought we had "taught" our patients that the trance belonged to them, when we debriefed them after treatment and listened carefully to *their* experiences we discovered that from their perspectives hypnosis was a two-person experience. Interestingly enough, patient belief in a two-person process carried over even to the self-hypnosis that we require of almost all our patients. They reported that they thought about us when they began their self-hypnosis, felt compliant with us when they did it or defiant of us on days when they did not do it, and even heard our voices when they did their own trance work between sessions.[1]

---

[1]There are three types of experience that we would call pure self-hypnosis. Some trances occur unintentionally, as when one is driving down a familiar highway, gets lost in thought, and does not pay conscious attention to what is going on around one, yet at some level is still aware enough not to drive off the road, have an automobile accident, or miss the turnoff. Unintentional trances also occur during aesthetic experiences, as when one goes to a play or concert that so enthralls one that 2 hours pass in a flash. We often use the term "mesmerized" to describe this type

The discussion so far should not be understood to mean that we see hypnosis in an old, authoritative way that implies that a powerful therapist "controls" a subject. Since we believe that effective communication requires entering the world of the patient and moving from there, it is questionable who is leading and who is following in this dance (see King et al., 1983, and Citrenbaum et al., 1985, for discussions of "pacing and leading"). The theoretical notion that hypnosis belongs to the therapeutic relationship and not to the subject alone has clinical implications that we will discuss in Chapter 4 when we explain the importance of "homework" and therapeutic directives.

So far, we have discussed what hypnosis is not. It is not an altered state of consciousness, or a sleeplike state, or something that belongs just to the subject. It is much harder to discuss what it is. Hypnosis is a very complex phenomenon. It can only be properly seen in the context of a relationship that itself is extremely fluid and complex. We are reminded of our favorite quote from the existential philosopher Friedrich Nietzsche (1954a, p. 530): "We no longer esteem ourselves sufficiently when we communicate ourselves. Our true experiences are not at all garrulous. They could not communicate themselves even if they tried. That is because they lack the right word. Whatever we have words for, that we have already gone beyond. In all talk there is a grain of contempt." Despite this limitation, and with as little contempt as possible, we will try to explain from an existential perspective what hypnotherapy is and why it is effective.

---

of self-hypnosis. The second type of pure self-hypnosis occurs when a person learns self-hypnosis from someone—often a professional—but practices it regularly long after the relationship with the teacher has ended. Over time the subject "owns" the self-hypnosis: it becomes disassociated from its original source. The third type of self-hypnosis is meditation. While many teachers of meditation like to claim that meditation and trance are fundamentally different, meditation does produce a trance experience. The intention of the experience may be different for a person practicing Zen meditation as opposed to a patient doing a prescribed self-hypnotic experience as part of his or her psychological or medical treatment, but both people still experience trances.

The complexity begins with an understanding that what hypnosis is and how and why it works differs for different subjects. Trance is a process, not a thing. For many patients the process of trance is similar to the working of a placebo drug in medicine. Many people in Western culture have notions about the power of hypnosis. They believe it can "cure" them; therefore it will, no matter how ineffectively the professional may use it. Many people suffer from behavioral habits they have had for many years. The reasons for establishing and maintaining these behaviors may be long gone, but these patients have told others and themselves they have no control over the behavior for so long that (1) they now believe it to be true and (2) it would be socially unacceptable (or seem so to them) to just stop the behavioral change because it implies to people in their life that they did have the power to end the behavior after all. Hypnotherapy then becomes the "cause" of the change that the patient was clearly ready to make before he or she made the therapy appointment. Hypnotherapy has two advantages here over traditional talking psychotherapy. First, because of social beliefs about the power of hypnosis, a faster "cure" is acceptable to the patient and to his or her family and friends. Second, there is less social stigma attached to the process of "being hypnotized" than there is to entering psychotherapy. Thus a wider range of persons, many of them unwilling to be treated conventionally, will use hypnosis. This process takes place, of course, almost always out of the patient's conscious awareness. They really do experience themselves as having no control over the behavior or symptom in question and they do believe that treatment did cure them—which it did. But in many cases hypnosis becomes a socially acceptable explanation of a behavioral change the patient was ready to make anyway.

We do not mean to suggest that the process of hypnotherapy is nothing more than an often effective placebo. On the contrary, we believe that hypnotherapy carried out by a skilled hypnotherapist can help many patients with a wide variety of problems. What we are suggesting here is that the process works differently for different patients, and we need to recognize that for *some* patients the most helpful part of the

treatment may be beliefs they themselves have about hypnosis before treatment even begins, or what we convey to
them about hypnosis near the beginning of our work with
them.[2] For some, the placebo effect by itself may lead to a
successful outcome. This explains why many unskilled professional hypnotherapists can honestly claim a 20–30% success rate, even for stubborn habits like cigarette smoking.

For many other patients the process of trance induction,
whether it be hypnotherapy in the office or directed self-
hypnosis between sessions, is part of a cooperative relationship between therapist and subject that becomes therapeutic
in nature. Most of this text will describe techniques that
enable patients to change beliefs, feelings, and behaviors in a
way that is healthier for them. While this process is complex
and different for each therapist–patient combination, it always
involves a focused attention by the subject[3] that requires him
or her "to be with" the experience in a fully present way, and
usually in a way different from his or her ordinary mode of
being-in-the-world. This presence is the tool the therapist can
then use within the context of the therapeutic relationship
to help the patient. How this presence is used depends on the
training and theoretical orientation of the therapist. One can
use language (suggestions) to help patients understand that
they are "capable of feats far beyond the range of what the
conscious ego imagines" (Hall, 1989, p. 5) or visual images
to alter the subjects' experience of themselves and their world.
The next chapter will discuss some of our specific views about
hypnosis such as types of inductions, depth of trance, and
susceptibility of subjects.

EXISTENTIAL THEORY

An attempt to do a complete overview of existential theory,
even in an introductory and superficial manner, is beyond the
scope of this text. Such a project would end up being a very

---

[2]We discuss this topic in more detail in the next chapter.
[3]Focused attention is the one hallmark of trances.

large text in and of itself. To date, we are not aware of any work that has attempted to summarize and integrate the major existential thinkers in philosophy, literature, psychology, and psychiatry. One of the major difficulties of presenting a complete summary of the thinking of all of the major existential writers is that there is so much disagreement among them. Unlike theories that center around the work of one person—Freudianism, for example—existentialism houses great diversity. It is, for example, the philosophic home of both religious writers and the man who proclaimed God to be dead. What we will do in this section is to describe some of the major existential principles that are the philosophic and theoretical underpinnings of our psychotherapeutic work, a major part of which includes the use of clinical hypnosis.

Coconstitutionality, Self-Concept, and Diagnostic Labeling

In Figure 1 (the popular "vase and faces" drawing) you can either view the center position as figure and the outside as ground, in which case you would see a vase, or you can treat the outer portion as figure and the center portion as ground, in which case you see faces. Or you can switch back and forth, as most people do, and see both. What you cannot do is make any meaning of the foreground without using the context or background. The background is as much a part of understanding the experience as the foreground. In a similar manner people and the world coconstitute each other. They shape the definition and meaning of each other. One does not and cannot exist without the other. They are in constant *dialogue* with each other. *Being* always means *being-in-the-world*. An attempt to understand a person separate from his or her world is an ontological mistake.

The concept of coconstitutionality has four major implications for understanding pathology and psychotherapy. One has to do with the notion of situated freedom, an idea discussed later in this chapter. The second has to do with how we understand any phenomena, including those believed to

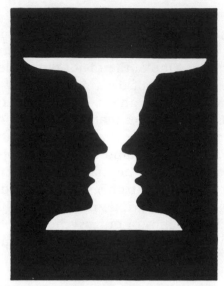

FIGURE 1. The "vase and faces" drawing.

be pathological. Most professionals see pathology as residing interdermally: for example, anxiety resides inside the skin of the anxious person either as a physiological reaction or as something inside the "psyche" of that person. An existentialist sees pathology (and all phenomena) as being located in and belonging to the dialectical relationship between the person and his or her world. This does not mean that the world is causing the problem, but rather that the subject is living in and responding to situations that call forth the response. Thus the pathology must be understood in that light.

The third idea related to coconstitutionality involves dealing with a person's self-concept and is perhaps the most radical departure from traditional Western thinking. In our culture, in which the basic philosophical model of understanding includes a person–world split (Descartes's subject–object split), one of the two basic psychological entities in the model is that which is variously called *I*, or *self*, or *ego*: a self-contained unit in some ways totally separate from the rest of the world. Because of this philosophical position shared by most thinking people in our culture, one of the most important and frequently asked questions in therapy is "Who am I?" One of the reasons many people come to therapy is because, as they would say it, "I have a negative self-concept." What this means is that the labels they have applied to themselves are not socially desirable ones. They think of themselves as ugly, uncreative, "bad," and so forth. Most therapists would see their job as trying to help such a person improve his or her self-concept or, to say it another way, to raise his or her self-esteem.

Existential thought suggests a different approach to understanding this problem in living. Existentialists would see the client's problem not in the answer to the question "Who am I?" but rather in the question itself. Existentialists would see the person as having "a problem" even if the answer was desirable, such as "I am smart" or "I am sexually attractive."

The question "Who am I?" calls for a thinglike answer, one that implies an objectlike consistency across situations. This consistency is only a reflection of the human condition that exists after one has alienated himself or herself from the world and sees the self as a thing. I can look at my pencil and ask "What is it?" I can answer "pencil" because it is an object and it will continue to be a pencil in all situations on my desk, in my hand, on the floor, and so on.

If human beings are in fact coconstituted by their world, then one could only begin to answer the question "Who am I?" by asking many more questions: "When?," "Where?," "With whom?," and so on. The answer to the question "Who am I?" depends as much on the situation as the person. For this reason psychiatric diagnostic labels are not taken too seriously by existential clinicians. For example, if a man were to come into our office complaining that he cannot have sex with his wife because he cannot maintain an erection, we could not label him as impotent without addressing the time, place, and person with whom he is impotent. Maybe 20 minutes of "therapy" with a prostitute would show him that he was not impotent. But at that point we could not switch and relabel him a potent man because he by himself is neither potent nor impotent (in fact *he by himself* does not exist, for he *always* exists within a situation). Potency is called forth by the dialogue between himself and his situation. In the same way a person sitting in the office is not by himself or herself a patient. He or she could only be a patient if the situation (in this case, the therapist) were willing to coconstitute him or her as patient. In this way, all psychiatric illnesses are partly made up by the family, friends, and doctors who are "helping."

We said before that a self-concept was problematic even if the specific concepts that constitute it seem desirable. For example, let us say that Jane feels intelligent. If it becomes important to her to have a concept of herself as intelligent, then she must do certain things. First, she must constantly work hard to keep achieving in areas that would support her concept of "Intelligent Jane" since her existence seems to be dependent on this self-definition in a very real psychological way. Second, she has to try to avoid all situations that might call this self-concept into question. Third, she will distort information that she receives when it is inconsistent with her already established self-concept. Carl Rogers (1947, p. 365) was one of the first to point this problem out when he wrote that "the Self-Concept resists assimilating into itself any percept which is inconsistent with its present organizations." This is true even if the new information is more positive in nature than the old concept. Everyone knows someone who has lost a lot of weight but cannot accept compliments because that person still "sees" himself or herself as a fat person. If a person has a concept of the self that he or she likes, that person will usually work hard to maintain that concept, that image, at all times. To accomplish this task, the person must negate the situational pole of the person–situation dialogue. Consequently, we get males, for example, who have a concept of themselves as independent (à la John Wayne) and try to remain "strong and independent" in all situations no matter how inauthentic that concept may be.

A therapist who is grounded in existential–phenomenological thought understands that the idea of a self-concept is one of the frequent forms in which alienation becomes manifest. The existential therapist will try to help clients give up the need to label themselves and to behave consistently according to that concept or label. The existential therapist will try to promote an alternative view of existence that encourages the person to remain in touch with how he or she experiences the world at any given moment and to let his or her constantly emerging needs and wants guide his or her behavior. *The sound of an ideal self-concept is silence.*

In Chapter 3, the first clinical chapter of this text, we explain how we use hypnotherapy to help clients "let go" of many things—anger, a painful history, excessive weight, and many more problems—but none more important than the need to label themselves.

The fourth implication that coconstitutionality has for therapy is the avoidance of using diagnostic labels. There are two reasons for this: First, as we mentioned above, this leads to negation of the situation (in the person–situation dialogue) which the labels imply. Second, an existentialist understands the nature of "being" such that being always includes "being-toward-a-future." By using a label, we lock a person into an actuality and negate future possibilities (for example, the possibility that next week he or she will not be schizophrenic). The effect of labeling was verified in a socially important study conducted by Rosenhan (1973). He sent eight students into mental hospitals where each one pretended to be disturbed during an initial interview; after this admission interview each student then acted in a normal manner. However, they were still identified as being "sick." Rosenhan (1973, p. 253) writes:

> A psychiatric label has a life and an influence of its own. Once the impression has been found that the patient is schizophrenic, the expectation is that he will continue to be schizophrenic. When a sufficient amount of time is passed, during which the patient has done nothing bizarre, he is considered to be in remission and available for discharge. But the label endures beyond discharge, with the unconfirmed expectation that he will behave as a schizophrenic again.

The Meaning of Anxiety

Most psychotherapy patients suffer from anxiety, either as a primary symptom or as a secondary symptom related to their problematic life. Hypnotherapy is a very effective treatment for anxiety. This is probably even more true for the caseloads of professionals who are known to use hypnosis in their practice. We have two beliefs about anxiety that influence our clinical work. William Fisher (1988) has done excellent phenomenological research on the meaning of anxiety. He found that anxiety almost always occurs when (1) an individual is called by his or her environment to perform; (2) the individual is unsure of his or her ability to do so; and (3) the outcome is important to him or her (usually more so than the situation calls for on the surface). Therefore, in psychotherapy we focus on the person–world dialogue to help the patient understand the meaning of his or her anxiety and deal with the roots of the patient's uncertainty about his or her abilities to perform in these situations.

Kierkegaard, often called the father of existential philosophy, states that "he who is schooled in anxiety is schooled in potentiality" (1954, p. 12) and also notes that "anxiety is always to be understood as oriented towards freedom" (1944, p. 38). Existentialists see anxiety as a calling card to the future. In today's uncertain world, people seem inordinately attached —almost in the manner of an addiction—to emotional safety, or more accurately, attached to the *illusion* of psychological safety. The great mass of people are running at full speed away from their existential dread and fear which is rooted in knowledge of the possibility of nonbeing. Today it seems that when the average person moves away from the sameness of everyday life, the accompanying anxiety becomes the cue for that person to (1) flee back to the sameness or (2) take a Valium. Kierkegaard calls this response to life the "shut-up personality." This is the reason so many couples, for example, stay in an unfulfilling relationship. A known misery seems better than the anxiety of the unknown. One potential explanation of the high incidence of drug (legal and illegal) abuse is its tranquilizing effect on anxiety, anxiety that is ontological in nature and that can never be stifled without paying a price. For more detailed discussion of this topic, see Rollo May's superb text, *The Meaning of Anxiety* (1977).

Because he or she understands the positive function of anxiety in human existence, the existential psychotherapist does two things. First, he or she helps the patient to relabel the meaning of anxiety. One of the biggest problems facing many patients, especially those who come from dysfunctional childhood homes, is a lack of knowledge about what "normal" is. When such people are faced with a task and are uncertain about their ability to perform in certain situations, they label their anxiety as a proof of their own inabilities and weaknesses and use this situation as one more opportunity to darken their self-image. It is important for the therapist to let these patients know that everyone feels anxiety at times. Only a person in total denial of feelings could dispute this truth. When patients see a person they label as brave or healthy they have the fantasy that these people do not suffer anxiety, that their hands never tremble, their bodies never perspire. They need to know that the difference between those seemingly healthy and brave persons, and the unhealthier ones, is that people in the first group see anxiety as "a calling card" and move ahead, after swallowing hard, because they are interested in seeing the results. Unhealthy people run away. The difference is in the response to anxiety, not the fact of it! Our patients often gain insight into themselves when we share some of our own experiences of anxiety and how we dealt with them. We do not intend to glorify anxiety— certainly, it does not feel good—but anxiety is not a sign in and of itself of pathology. Patients need to be encouraged to move forward in the face of anxiety and should be supported and congratulated for every small step they make in this regard. Patients should also know that what they may call anxiety, others may call excitement and make efforts (such as gambling or entering into risky business ventures) to experience.

The other important thing a hypnotherapist can do is teach patients techniques to reduce anxiety to a manageable level. These include dual hypnotic techniques for use in the office and self-hypnotic techniques for use at home. (These techniques will be discussed elsewhere in this text.) One significant difference between existentially oriented therapists and other therapists is that we teach patients to manage their reaction to anxiety, but we never attempt to eliminate the feeling of anxiety as a treatment goal because that would doom the therapy to failure: death is the only total anxiety reducer life has to offer. We hope to teach patients to value their anxiety. As Rollo May (1981, p. 19) writes, "After many a therapeutic hour, which I would call successful, the client leaves with more anxiety than when he came in; only now the anxiety is conscious rather than unconscious, constructive rather than destructive." Or as Nietzsche (1954b, p. 129) said, "One must still have chaos in oneself to be able to give birth to a dancing star."

Freedom, Responsibility, and the "They"

Philosophers and social scientists who belong to the existential school differ about many specific beliefs. For example, some existential philosophers believe in God, while others argue that God is dead. The one thing all existential thinkers have in common is faith in the reality of *human freedom*. This faith is central to the belief system and clinical work of all existentialists. As Warnock (1970, p. 1) states at the beginning of his often-cited book, *Existentialism*:

> The aim, above all, to show people *that they are free*, to open their eyes to something which has always been true, but which for one reason or another may have not always have been recognized, namely, that men are free to choose, not only what to do on a specific occasion but what to value and how to live. The readers of existential philosophy are being asked, not merely to consider the nature of human freedom, but to *experience* freedom and to practice it. (emphasis in original)

Rollo May (1989, p. 19), in his recently revised text, *The Art of Counseling*, states, "Freedom is a basic principle, in fact a sine quo non, of personality. It is by this characteristic that we separate human beings from animals." Jean-Paul Sartre

(1966, p. 26) says, "The indispensable fundamental condition of all action is the freedom of the agent."

Patients frequently argue that their behavior has consequences, often dramatic or severe ones, and therefore it does not seem to them that their choices are always free. Earlier in this chapter we talked about how people in the world coconstitute each other. All choices are made in the world, in a context or situation, and therefore all choices have consequences, sometimes known and sometimes unknown. This fact does not negate free will. It is naive to believe that free will means freedom from consequences for your decisions. Choices are sometimes limited by physical realities. If you are in jail, for example, you may not be free to chose to go to a baseball game, but, even in such a situation there are still choices to make. One could choose to get depressed about the situation or to spend each night reading, reflecting, and growing from the experience. The fact that all choices are not available at a given moment does not mean one does not have freedom: existential freedom must always be understood to occur within a situation with consequences and some physical limitations.

One of the first detailed discussions of the value of honoring your freedom and taking responsibility for your life appears in Homer's "The Myth of Orestes" in *The Odyssey* (1967). Orestes is the grandson of Atreus, whose family was cursed after a power struggle with the gods. Orestes's mother, Clytemnestra, kills his father. Greek civil law requires Orestes to kill his father's slayer but Greek religious law defines matricide as a sin. Orestes finally kills his mother and is then visited by the Furies, punitive spirits sent by the gods. After years of suffering he asks the gods for relief. Apollo is appointed as his spokesman at the trial. When Apollo tells the gods that Orestes is not to blame given his impossible situation, Orestes stands up and takes responsibility for his actions.

We cannot overemphasize to patients the therapeutic value of accepting their freedom. *Recovery from all disorders begins when one sees oneself as a volunteer in, rather than a victim of, the situation.* We begin psychotherapy by making subtle changes in the patient's language. We encourage our patients to use "I" (to own one's beliefs) rather than the generic "people" and to say "I *chose* to" rather than "I *have* to." As soon as people can begin to see how their choices put them in their present situation they can begin to truly have hope that they can learn to make choices that will change the situation. This is the beginning of the therapeutic process.

Can we be absolutely sure in some God-given metaphysical sense that freedom is a true characteristic of the human condition? Is freedom just our illusion or delusion? No one will ever know for sure in this lifetime; however, even if belief in human freedom is only an illusion, it is the most helpful of all possible illusions. No matter how bad things get, there will always be a hope for a way out based on one's own actions rather than wishing for others to help. There is less chance of feeling "stuck" with this belief system.

Since on the surface it sounds so logical and healthy to experience one's self as free, why doesn't everyone think that way all the time? Why is it that the most pervasive psychological theory in modern Western culture, behaviorism, says that we share the basic characteristics of an earthworm, a pigeon, and a laboratory rat and that the study of such animals teaches us much about ourselves? Because freedom has an inescapable accomplice, what Kierkegaard calls "dread responsibility." Responsibility is the child of freedom. Many people try to abort this child by pretending that it does not exist for them. This is what Sartre (1966) called "living in bad faith." Sartre said that when we are confronted with the freedom to do and to think whatever we chose, we inevitably suffer anguish. He says we often are unable to bear the thought of a boundless freedom. In order to escape from that anguish, we adopt a cover of bad faith, pretending to be not as free as we really are. This is what existentialists call "inauthentic living."

Almost any experienced psychotherapist who has confronted a patient with his or her own freedom will already understand this concept. Often patients reveal an obvious anguish when they begin to struggle with the notion of being responsible for their condition. Some even leave therapy because ongoing depression or some other symptom seems easier to bear than the weight of responsibility.

Moshe Talmon (1990, p. 5), who recently published fascinating research on the outcomes of a single psycho-therapy session, states that "therapists should also be aware of the powerful potential therapeutic effects both of telling the patient that he must take responsibility for his own life, and of reasuring him that he can manage without therapeutic help." We do not intend to suggest that no one really needs psychotherapy, or that all people need is the correct attitude. But we do believe that therapists should never underestimate the powerful effect of owning one's life. As Willie Nelson sings in his well-known song "Black Rose," "The devil made me do it the first time, the second time I done it on my own." This "macho" attitude promotes recovery a lot faster than the "I'm addicted" or "I'm the child of an alcoholic so what can you expect" attitude.

As Rollo May (1977, p. 47) states in *The Meaning of Anxiety*, "The courageous man prefers, when ill, to have it said, 'This is not fate, this is guilt.' For then *his possibility of doing something about his condition is not removed from him*"[4] (our emphasis).

When we teach this material in professional workshops the first question that usually comes up is, "What about those disorders where the patient seemingly has no responsibility, such as biological disorders or the developmental results of such severe childhood problems as sexual abuse?" Even here the patient needs to own responsibility to begin treatment. Psychiatric disorders that are generally believed to be mostly biological in nature, such as schizophrenia and major mood disorders, do not respond well to hypnotic treatment, and therefore are not within the scope of this text. We do believe, however, that even these patients are responsible for their own response to their disorder and its treatment. Every thera-pist has had experience with patients with manic–depressive

[4]In this quote May uses the term "guilt" in the Kierkegaardian sense of "responsibility."

disorder who respond to medication but who periodically reduce or stop their medication (probably because it feels good at first to experience a manic high) and who thereafter require a hospital admission. It is not the illness that stops someone from taking his or her medication; rather, the person himself or herself *chooses* not to take the medication. Likewise, some biologically depressed people "force" themselves out of the house and work to break the cycle of depression while others give in to the vaguest hint of a "blue mood."

In terms of the history of a severe negative environmental impact, such as childhood abuse, the therapist, while affirming that the patient was not to blame for the abuse and while expressing sympathy for the helpless child, must let the adult patient know that now he or she has choices to make about how to interpret and respond to a history of abuse. Two people could have the exact same history. One might believe, to paraphrase Nietzsche, "that which does not kill me makes me stronger," while the other may walk around for the rest of his or her life with the face of a victim. Each person is responsible for understanding and using his or her own history toward making a recovery. As Mary Catherine Bateson (1991) says, we have multiple versions of the same experience. It is not that one is a true remembrance and another is false, but rather that sometimes one thing is emphasized in memory and other times the emphasis changes.

To demonstrate this point, Bateson asked one of the authors (King) to understand his life as a logical series of events leading up to the present. He remembered being the eldest son in a Jewish family, programmed for the professional and monetary success he now enjoys, the value he holds regarding education, the way he values and behaves toward his children, and so on. It all seemed logical and clear. Then Bateson directed him to understand his life as a series of chance events that led to his present state. He remembered wanting to be a medical doctor but not being able to pass chemistry. At the same time he had a great teacher in an introductory psychology class, and as a consequence became a psychology major. Later he thought about how he stumbled into a continuing education hypnosis course (he was really interested in the study of consciousness, not clinical skills) that was offered on his only free night of the week, and of the lucky series of events that all had to happen for him to meet his future wife, and so on. Obviously, the same history can be understood in a number of different ways depending upon the intent and emphasis of the analysis of self-analysis.

Being responsible also means learning to stop respond-ing to the tyranny of the "They." Heidegger's term is one of our favorite philosophic phrases because it is so self-explana-tory: as soon as we say it to patients they grin and seem to intuitively understand its meaning. As children we all are encouraged to work hard and be responsible to please the "They" as if somehow this generalized approval of everybody seems to matter. Too many of us give up true pleasure, re-fusing to raise our voices in anger even when justified, and in general strive to be such good people because, after all, the "They" expect it even if it takes a psychological toll. Nietzsche (1954b, p. 282) says, "At bottom, these simpletons want a single thing most of all: that nobody should hurt them. Thus, they try to please and gratify everybody. This, however, is cowardness, even if it is to be called virtue." Existential psy-chotherapists can help patients to see the folly of working hard just to please other people. A person is responsible to himself or herself for his or her life, not to the group to sup-port its standards. As Warnock (1970, p. 20) notes, "One essential for the morally adult man is to create his own sys-tem of values and to reject the stock morality of his group."

To live a healthy life one does not need to reject the values of the "They" just for the sake of rejecting them. In fact, it is quite compatible with healthy living to accept many group values. The important issue is how free one feels to accept or reject any position or belief based on one's own perceptions of the world as opposed to feeling pressured by others to believe or behave a certain way—or worse yet, not even knowing that one has that choice. The voice of the "They" is often experienced as a given in life, like gravity. Sartre (1962) says that the man who unthinkingly accepts his condition, including the values he lives by, as if it were inevitable is living in bad faith; but people who know they can live by any values they choose and decide actively to abide by the traditional moral code are not living in bad faith. Sometimes it is difficult at first glance to distinquish between a person living in good or bad faith the therapist will need to probe these issues since an existence lived in bad faith is often at the root of the psychological issues that prompt the patient to seek treatment.

The Will to Power

If responsibility for oneself is the beginning of recovery, the feeling of having increased personal power and potency is the ultimate successful outcome of all psychotherapy. Most of the hypnotic techniques described later in this text are aimed at the development and enhancement of power and potency. In fact, we originally intended to subtitle this book "Theory and Techniques for the Will to Power." How one exercises his or her personal power is probably more a moral than a therapeutic issue; however, there can be no doubt that believing oneself to be the director of one's own movie is psychologically healthy.

We believe that the philosophic work that probably has the most important insights for psychotherapy is Nietzsche's *Thus Spake Zarathustra* (1954b). Here Nietzsche, through Zarathustra, speaks eloquently of human development toward the higher man (often called the "superman"), who is similar to Maslow's (1971) self-actualized individual. He speaks clearly and often about the need to exercise personal power:

> Where I found the living, there I found the will to power. (1954b, p. 226)

> Willing liberates: that is the true teaching of will and liberty. (1954b, p. 199)

> Do whatever you will, but first be such as are able to will! (1954b, p. 284)

Matthew Fox, the popular theologian, in an interview in *Psychology Today* (1989) states, "I think psychology is in danger of making a mistake similar to the one made by the church when it focuses on the question, 'What is your problem?' It should ask, 'What is your power?'"

Moshe Talmon (1990) has recently done pioneering work on single-session psychotherapy. He concludes that the essence of successful single-session psychotherapy is the empowerment of the patient by the therapist. He believes it is critical for patients to receive the congruent messages, "I believe in you" and "I believe in your ability."

The will to power has two different meanings for psychotherapy. The first meaning is that a person who experiences a sense of empowerment has a major say in his or her own life. The second meaning is literally willpower. For many professionals this character trait is often overlooked and not necessarily encouraged. Sometimes when a patient refuses to work hard on recovery by using any of his or her willpower therapists excuse that condition by pathologizing it and calling it an addiction. Mental and physical health requires a prolonged and persistent effort by each individual. It is the job of the therapist to convey this message consistently to the client, to use every persuasive means possible to let the patient know that recovery is possible, but that it will require hard work by the patient himself or herself. All patients also need to know that *they* gain the rewards of that good work or have to bear the consequences of lack of effort.

Probably because we teach professional workshops on hypnotherapy both of us have treated a large number of psychotherapists. As one can tell from reading this book, our previous published works are characterized more by common sense than by brilliance. Often fellow professionals who become our patients say to us, "Your books are good but we could have written them too." We respond, "That's right— you *could* have, but we *did*. That's why you paid to sit in on a workshop while we were getting paid to teach it." One's place in life is not decided by lottery, but rather by hard work. If one only painted what was easy, the Sistine Chapel might still be beige and we would never have heard of Michelangelo. Both of us have worked with individual professional athletes, as well as with professional teams. The average person would be surprised to learn how hard these people with "natural gifts" work at their trade. Football is a Sunday sport only to the fans.

It is important for patients to realize that they must do what they must do. Heart and lungs do not care how hard it is to stop smoking: they only respond if one stops or not. Carl Jung (1964, p. 29) notes in his introduction to an important beginning Zen book, "Zen demands intelligence and will-power, as do all the greater things which desire to become real." Hermann Hesse (1951), talking through his character Siddhartha, who is speaking to a friend, says that his strength lies in his ability to think, wait, and fast. The fasting in this phrase represents willpower, which combined with intelligence and patience is Hesse's formula for personal power.

Existential Uncertainty

When one of us was 5 years old, he had a pet rabbit that kept escaping from his yard and eventually had to be taken to the zoo. Every week that summer he and his father would visit the zoo and visit the cage with 50 to 100 rabbits in it. Each week the child would ask, "Which is mine?" Each week his father would point to a nearby rabbit and say, "There he is!" His father's action made the child feel very happy. But here is the catch: a child grows up in a world where it becomes very difficult to believe he knows where his rabbit is. Usually, in the long term, attempts to falsely simplify the world end up slapping you in the face. For short-term treatment of some symptoms it is possible (and sometimes even desirable) to alter the patient's reality system to a clear belief that can promote needed change. For growth in long-term treatment, however, patients must always struggle to accept the complex, and to some degree unknowable, facets of human existence. An existentialist therapist encourages openness to the unknown and the ability to let go of preconceptions and any "need to know" during long-term psychotherapy and hypnotherapy. The hypnotherapy we do is not insight-oriented in terms of discovering the "causes" of personal problems. In fact, we usually ask our clients during intake if they would be willing to get better without knowing why they had the problem or how the hypnosis works. Only three people have ever said no.

Existential moments in life do not have a why: they just are. Hypnotherapy can help people let go of the clinging to simple "truths" that often functionally limit the number of options they experience. As Hermann Hesse so wisely said,

> "Clarity" and "truth" are words that we often hear used side by side, as if they meant more or less the same thing. Yet they stand for entirely different things! Rarely, very rarely is the truth clear, and even more rarely is clarity true! The truth is almost always complex, obscure, and ambiguous— every statement, especially a "clear" statement—does it violence. . . . Maxims are charming, they are useful, educational, witty, informative—but they are never true. Because the opposite of every maxim is also true. (1974, p. 94)

The existential novelist Milan Kundera, best known for *The Unbearable Lightness of Being*, describes a good novel in much the same words we would use to describe a good psychotherapist:

> A novel does not assert anything; a novel searches and imposes questions. . . . The stupidity of people comes from having an answer for everything. When Don Quixote went out into the world, that world turned into a mystery before his eyes. That is the legacy of the first European novel to the entire subsequent history of the novel. The novelist teaches the reader to comprehend the world as a question. There is wisdom and tolerance in that attitude. (1981, p. 237)

This chapter has not been intended to be a complete review of existential philosophy or psychology, but was designed to highlight some of the important insights from this school of thought that underline the clinical work we do, specifically our style of hypnotherapy.

CHAPTER 2

Existential Hypnosis

The past 250 years have produced many definitions of hypnosis and trance. The earlier definitions tended to make the process into something unusual and mysterious. For example, in a popular early text, Carpenter (1900) said that trance was "an abnormal state of the mind and body induced by special methods, the outcome of which is a class of phenomena differing essentially from ordinary human experience." Gavitz (1991) details the history of trances from ancient time, beginning more than 4,000 years ago in China. Some of the more modern definitions tend to sound scientific, using phrases such as "dissociative state," "altered state of consciousness," or "sociocognitive alteration of perception." In truth, however, neither the researchers who study hypnosis nor the theorists who write about this phenomenon have come to a reasonable consensus about what hypnosis is. After centuries of observing trancelike behaviors professionals in the field cannot even agree as to whether hypnotized subjects can behave in nonordinary ways or, as Spanos (1991, p. 324) believes, whether these behaviors "are fundamentally similar to other more modern forms of social action and can be accounted for without recourse to special psychological states or processes."

While this lack of agreement concerning even the basic issues about hypnosis and trance poses interesting dilemmas for the researcher or theorist, it is of little concern to the clinician with an existential orientation. For such therapists the important data for their work are the experiences of the client; rarely do these experiences relate to the issues that academics (including ourselves) are so preoccupied with. Patients generally care little whether trance is truly an altered state, whether the neodisassociative model is an accurate description, and so on. For most patients, trance is whatever they believe it to be, which is mostly *what the therapists tells them it is.* The communication about trance that takes place between the clinician and the patient is more important than specific "facts" about hypnosis such as whether Erickson's use of indirect suggestion is better than Spiegel's more direct approach.

PATIENTS' BELIEFS ABOUT HYPNOSIS

The key to effective existential hypnosis is the therapist–patient dialogue, and especially what is communicated *about* hypnosis and what is communicated *during* hypnosis. For example, patients came to our office feeling stuck and complaining that their ordinary ways of getting unstuck have not worked. Consequently, whatever one thinks of Spanos's (1991) argument that trance behaviors are quite ordinary, it is important to assure patients that hypnosis will give them a superordinary ability to solve their problems. In fact, when the patient "buys" into this idea, you have communicated the first important "hypnotic" message of your therapy. It does not really matter what your beliefs about the nature of hypnosis are so long as you yourself believe that this process will help the patient and so long as you can communicate your belief in its therapeutic effect to your patients.

Obviously this discussion simplifies a complex phenomenon belief system. The reader might ask, If it is this simple, why don't we just tell patients they will get better after one hypnotic session? Indeed, experienced hypnotherapists have seen examples of patients with seemingly complex and long-standing problems, such as sexual dysfunction or habit disorders, get better literally overnight as a result of hypnosis. Yet, because of psychodynamics such as a symptom's secondary gains, most patients require some effort before significant improvement is noted. As Yapko (1990, p. 418) says in *Trancework* while speaking about a symptom's function and associated secondary gains, "If these two issues are not adequately addressed, directly or indirectly, success in treatment is virtually impossible." It would set people up for failure to give them an early expectation of a "miracle" cure. Promoting fast "cures" could also negate the vital therapeutic message that persistence and determination are important in life. However, when one of these one-session cures does occur, we are not surprised. On the contrary, we smile so the patient will believe we expected it all along and therefore they can trust its reality.

The second belief that existential hypnotherapists need to convey to new patients is that they can go into a trance and that trance is a safe and comfortable experience. Before we do trance work we give the patient what we call our "2-cent, 2-minute hypnosis lecture." It goes something like this:

"Now, Frank, there are three issues I want to tell you about trance or hypnosis. First, trance is a normal, natural experience, it is something you do everyday, but you just don't call it trance. For example, you drive down a familiar road or a boring road like a turnpike and get so lost in thought that the next thing you are aware of is that you are 5 miles farther down the road than you last noted, yet you haven't missed your turnoff or had an accident because some part of you was monitoring the road all along. We call this 'highway hypnosis' or 'turnpike trance.' Maybe you remember going to a show or concert that so mesmerized you that when it was over you looked at your watch because you could not believe 2 hours had passed: it seemed more like 15 minutes. So the first thing I want to tell you is that trance is a natural experience that may disappoint you because most people expect dramatics—a sleeplike or a druglike experience. You will lean back in that chair and probably feel more relaxed than now, but you will continue to hear me talk, and probably about 10 minutes into the experience say, 'It's not working!' If you have a strong ego, you'll blame me and say I'm a bad hypnotist. If you have a weak ego, you'll blame yourself and say you're a bad subject. Now I have some ways to let you know it's working that I'll share later on, but I can assure you while the experience may disappoint you, the results won't. And after all, results are why you're here, not just to have a neat experience.

"Second, Frank, I want you to know that anyone can go into a trance, with two exceptions—hyperactive kids or retarded citizens. Now, Frank, you have been here already for 40 minutes and I'm leaping to the clinical conclusion that your attention span is at least 2 minutes and your I.Q. at least 70, so there is no doubt about your ability to experience trance. Some people will be able to follow any instructions I suggest, and for other people I have to fish around for specific methods that match their cognitive style—but that just determines how hard I have to work.

"Third, I want to let you know that trance is the ultimate in self-control: you will always be in control. In fact, [name the patient's symptom] has you out of control and this technique will give you more control. People often ask me questions such as, 'What happens if I have a heart attack while they are in trance?' I tell them, 'You'll hear me moan, "Come out of trance, and call 911." Since we're in Pittsburgh they will put you on hold, but that will be my problem.' Many women think, and some ask, 'What would happen if you made a sexual advance while you have me in trance?' I answer, 'I would never do that, but if I did what I do know about trance tells me that the result would be the same as if I made the advance now.' The trance won't help me gain any power over them or you.

"So, in summary, trance is a normal, natural experience, one that I know you can do and that will give you even more control, not take it from you. Any questions?"

The third thing that patients must believe for hypnotherapy to work is that they have actually been in a trance. We convince them of this truth in a number of ways. First, as soon as patients alert themselves, we ask, "About how long does it seem since you first closed your eyes?" Over 80% of the time even light-trance subjects reveal significant time distortions—often a report of 10, 15, or 20 minutes, when it has actually been 45 to 50 minutes. We then show them how much time has passed and let them know how time distortion is a predictible trance phenomenon and proof of how well they have done, especially for the first session. Second, we point out physical stillness, slowed breathing, and other trance indicators to confirm that they have experienced trance. We call these indicators "trance convincers" or "trance ratifiers."

What the patient believes about trance is far more important then what academics in the field have to say about this phenomenon. If patients believe that hypnosis can help them, if they believe that they can be hypnotized, and later if they believe that they were in fact in a trance, the clinician is set up to do good clinical work. These beliefs are not the work itself, but the grounding for it.

HYPNOSIS AND PSYCHOTHERAPY

As we said before, *the therapist–patient dialogue or relationship is the most important variable of hypnotherapy.* Everything else can only be understood in the context of this relationship. This relationship is what Shor (1959, p. 585) called "the flesh and blood of hypnosis." Mason (1960, p. 24) called the hypnotist–subject relationship "the most fundamental of all hypnotic phenomena."[1] The personal characteristics and professional training required of a good hypnotherapist are the same as those required of any good psychotherapist. These personal traits include intelligence, flexibility, analytical thinking, empathy, sensitivity, and an ability to be in deeply intimate relationships. In addition, we believe that hypnotherapists must also be able to trust the trance process and use the process themselves. In terms of professional training, we believe in a solid grounding in normal developmental pro-

[1] These two references (1959 and 1960) are old for a 1990s book; however, Shor and Mason succinctly but eloquently say what we believe and what many more recently published works conclude.

cesses,[2] an understanding of psychodynamics, and supervised training in a number of types of psychotherapy. We believe that hypnosis is only one technique to be used in psychotherapy, hopefully by a skilled therapist with many techniques at his or her disposal to use as needed. An old study (Moss, Riggen, Coyne, & Bishop, 1965) yet to be replicated suggests that therapists who use hypnosis regularly received less formal training in psychotherapy as well as less personal psychotherapy for themselves. If it is true that the therapist who uses hypnosis is less trained than the psychotherapist who emphasizes other techniques, this is a sad commentary on hypnotherapy. Good existential therapists must pay attention to the gestalt of the therapy relationship process and recognize that hypnosis is only one tool of their trade. Hypnotherapy should not be the treatment of choice for everyone; even when it is, it rarely should be the entire treatment. Even what happens inside the trance work (metaphorically speaking) is psychotherapy and requires an understanding of development, psychodynamics, and pathology—not just knowledge of techniques.

The two biggest misunderstandings of the work of Milton Erickson are that (1) he made up magic metaphors as his only technique, and (2) he only used hypnosis. First, he did not limit himself to using metaphors with patients. He had a good background in traditional psychiatry and worked very hard to understand each person's symptoms in the context of his or her life and then developed a treatment plan for that person (Hammond, 1988). Second, as Lawrence Kirmayer noted (1988, p. 157), "A great many of Erickson's cases did not involve hypnosis in any conventional sense. . . . Erickson's most important contributions are not techniques, but

---

[2]We believe that too few therapists are grounded enough in the theory of normal development. Some of the interventions that Milton Erickson reports that seem so mysterious to many therapists are little more than applied "common sense" if one takes normal developmental principles and expectations into account. Erickson urged his students to spend time studying the normal family at the circus, in the supermarket, and elsewhere, especially for learning about clinical work with children.

changes in the values or ethics under which psychotherapy is conducted."

In every workshop we teach we are asked about the ethics of hypnosis as if hypnosis raised ethical problems different from other professional techniques. The ethics of hypnosis should be the same as one's professional ethics. For example, the two of us do not identify ourselves as hypnotherapists, but rather as psychologists who often use hypnotherapy in our clinical work. The ethics we subscribe to are the ethics of our field (the American Psychological Association), especially as it refers to psychotherapy. So, even though we can help patients with pain control, we will not try to fill their dental cavities, for neither of us is trained or licensed to do so. Likewise, a dentist should not be helping his or her patients with weight control or in dealing with the fear of flying, even if he or she is skilled at trance inductions.

HYPNOTIZABILITY

As we said before, existentialists believe that all hypnotic phenomena can only be understood in the context of the therapist–patient relationship. Let us begin by discussing the popular, and usually misunderstood, concept of hypnotizability.

We offer this analogy. Everyone has the ability to write poetry. Clearly, some people are naturally more poetic than others. Whether it is a gift they are born with or a learned phenomenon is questionable. What is not questionable is the notion of individual difference in ability to be poetic. Yet, given the proper environment—stimulation, encouragement, training, and the like—everyone can create something poetic. Also, even the most gifted poet can have his or her ability stifled given a harsh and anxious environment. Likewise, as Diamond (1984, p. 3) notes, "Some capacity for hypnotic trance experience resides within the repertoire of most, if not all, persons." Thus, in most cases, the hypnotherapist provides an environment and an opportunity that encourages each individual patient to "let go" and experience trance.

As existentialists, we understand all human character-istics as a process, not a "state" or "trait." The process of going in and out of trance, like any other human process, is part of the dialogue between the person and his or her world. It is the interaction between the natural trance abilities of the subject (which admittedly vary greatly from subject to subject) and the environment at any given moment, especially the relationship between the subject and the hypnotist, that deter-mines the ability to do trance. It is the job of the professional to be skilled and flexible enough to provide what each per-son needs to facilitate his or her trance abilities—whatever those abilities may be. Most patients require a trusting rela-tionship with their therapist in which they feel safe enough to experience trance and a belief that it will be helpful for them to engage in the trance experience with their hypno-therapist. Beyond these essentials, there are many individual differences in terms of what is needed by each patient. Some patients respond better to a direct, almost "authoritarian" approach, while others require an indirect, permissive, natu-ralistic induction. Some need a structured induction ("Close your eyes and imagine a chalkboard with the number 50," and so on), while others do best with an informal conversa-tional induction. Some patients require an established rela-tionship with the therapist, while others are raring to go when they first sit down. There is no right way to do trance, only ways that are effective for each patient; the best approach may vary over time, even with the same patient. We have both had the experience of patients who at first seem very "non-susceptible" but after time passed, as our therapeutic relation-ship developed, they were able to allow themselves to use trance to help them achieve their therapeutic ends.

SUSCEPTIBILITY

A number of tests of hypnotizability or susceptibility have been developed and popularized. Most notable are the Stan-ford Scale (Weitzenhoffer & Hilgard, 1959), the Harvard Scale

(Shor & Orne, 1962), and the Spiegel Induction Profile (Spiegel, 1974). These tests are all made up of items measuring responses to direct suggestion, for example, directions to raise or lower an arm or to sway. These tests do not measure a subject's potential to respond to nonauthoritarian and indirect approaches (see Barber, 1980); more importantly, they do not (and cannot) account for motivational factors.

We believe that if a patient is in enough pain, whether emotional or physical, and comes to believe that hypnosis will help relieve his or her suffering, the patient will inevitably become "susceptible." Michael Diamond (1987) reports a case of a young woman who scored consistently low on a variety of hypnotizability tests given as part of an experiment. He claims that she would have been labeled "refractory to hypnosis" or "untrainable." He then began to work with her in a clinical manner (which presumably meant that the hypnosis work had relatively more meaning for her than when it was just part of an experiment). She was then able to use autohypnotic experiences, reported as having reached a profound depth of trance. Zahourek (1990) found that some patients at Denver General Hospital achieved successful trance states when they were experiencing pain, but lost their ability to enter trance as they recovered and were in less need of it. His conclusion, like ours, is that "patient motivation is crucial."

We are not suggesting that no individual differences in the ability of patients to use trance for their therapeutic ends exist: such differences obviously do exist. Likewise, patients manifest individual differences in their abilities to use psychotherapy in general to meet their needs. We would never give someone a "therapy ability" test before beginning work with them because we believe that everyone can be helped to some degree by the psychotherapy process. For the same reasons we would never use a hypnotizability scale with a clinical patient. As existentialists, we know that the most important factor in our work is the patient's belief system. If we utilized a scale we would be required to engage in some form of "therapeutic fiction": we would have to tell each patient who asked about susceptibility that he or she was highly susceptible. To do otherwise, we would create a negative self-fulfilling prophecy. We also believe that the problematic consequences that accompany this negative belief about the patient's trance ability are partly a function of the therapist being "hypnotized" into believing in the patient's "lack of ability" and not working as hard as he or she needs to.

There are three keys to successful trance use within a psychotherapy context. First, convince each patient that hypnosis will help him or her and that he or she does have the ability to use it. Second, recognize that some people are ready to begin hypnosis work as soon as they enter your office while others need to develop trust in the therapeutic relationship first. The therapist must allow for such individual differences. Third, be flexible. By this we mean that some patients need a formal, structured, or authoritarian induction, while others need a more informal naturalistic approach; some patients need an emphasis on hypnosis work led by the clinician, while others need an emphasis on their self-hypnosis work; and some patients bore easily and need the therapist to constantly change the induction, while others respond better to a familiar routine.

LEVEL OF TRANCE

There has been a lot of discussion—indeed, too much discussion—in the professional hypnosis literature about the level of trance subjects go into and what the implications of these levels are for treatment. Over the years many scales have been developed to measure trance depth. These scales have anywhere from 5 to 50 divisions, ranging from the "insusceptible" to the "profoundly somnambulistic." Such scales may have some research value (the operative word is *may*) but they have little clinical value to an existential hypnotherapist. In practice, we find the concept of "depth of trance" to be harmful because too many beginning therapists are themselves "hypnotized" by this idea and spend too much clinical time trying to deepen an already workable trance experience. These efforts waste valuable clinical time and give the patient the wrong message, for the therapist's struggle to deepen the trance beyond the patient's natural style promotes the message that the patient is not yet ready to do the needed clinical work. We try to convey the exact opposite message to our patients. Remember, as existentialists we see our main job as altering the patient's belief system from one in which the patient sees himself or herself as "stuck" to one in which he or she sees himself or herself ready for change.

We have made three valuable observations regarding level of trance and clinical work. First, each patient seems to have a "natural" depth of trance that he or she can go into more often and more easily. This natural depth is probably related to the person's cognitive style and personality characteristics, which in turn interact with the style of the hypnotist and the level of trust the patient has in the process. Degrees of natural depth of trance are much too complex to be predictable; however, once you have worked with a patient in trance a few times you can predict what depth of trance he or she is likely to go into.

Second, there is an ebb and flow to the trance experience. Since it is a process, not a static state, patients will often lighten and deepen the trance during the course of a single therapeutic session. This is another reason it makes no sense to try to measure depth of trance because by the time this measurement is recorded the subject may have shifted depth. Some of these shifts in depth have clinical implications, so the therapist needs to pay attention. For example, when patients get frightened by an internal experience during a session they will often either lighten the trance and become restless or deepen the trance in ways that a carefully trained observer can notice. Some days patients are just not ready to do trance work, and so they will not allow themselves to let go and have their normal trance experience. On the other hand, many times the shifting trance depths during a session or the patient's change in depth experiences from one session to the next occur seemingly without reason. If a patient inquires about this phenomenon and together we seem to be without a clue, we just tell them, "That's the way it is!" We believe that existential moments in life do not always have a why—

they just are. Accepting this "fact" is a major goal of all psychotherapy with an existential orientation.

The third, and by far the most important, observation about level of trance is that it rarely matters for clinical work. All of the techniques we will present in this text seem to work equally well for patients, no matter what level of trance they as individuals can achieve.[3] In our professional training workshops in hypnotherapy we often have many medical people in attendance and therefore usually do a section on hypnotic control of pain and bleeding. The demonstration we use involves inserting a 20-gauge needle through a vein in the back of the hand. (This is a sensitive area—just pinch it to see—and the needle is relatively thick, so this can be an impressive demonstration.) We usually use three or four subjects per demonstration. Some people will not let us get near them with the needle unless they are in a deep somnambulistic trance. Other subjects achieve such a light trance that only a well-trained observer would label this experience a trance; yet each of these subjects can achieve an equal degree of pain reduction and control over bleeding when we remove the needle.

The goal in hypnotherapy is not depth of trance, but reduction in the presenting symptoms. Therapists need to stop worrying so much about "how deep the patient goes under" and begin to respect the natural idiosyncratic style of each

---

[3]There are two exceptions: The first exception is patients who have suffered trauma early in life, such as sexual or physical abuse, and who are using hypnotherapy to remember and work through this type of experience. These patients often (not always) need to achieve a moderately deep trance in order to do this work. Since these patients often have dissociative abilities anyway, deep trance is usually a naturally occurring event. When it is not, we recommend that a good therapeutic relationship be established before the trance work begins and that time be taken for nonthreatening trance training before the clinical work begins. The second exception is patients who require hypnoanesthesia for surgical procedures (when ordinary anesthetic agents are contraindicated). The deep or somnambulistic trance necessary for such patients may only be achievable by 10–15% of the population.

patient, constantly letting patients know that now that they have achieved trance they can begin to look forward to the personal growth they came into hypnotherapy to achieve.

THE "HOW" OF HYPNOTIC INDUCTIONS

If you can effectively master three principles we will discuss in a moment, doing hypnotic inductions is quite easy. The difficult part is doing the clinical work after the trance is induced. For this reason, hypnotherapists must first be trained psychotherapists. Many professionals regard "lay" hypnotists as dangerous. We do not see anything dangerous about the trance experience. The biggest danger related to use of hypnosis by untrained persons (or unskilled professionals) is that they will be ineffective. The danger therein is that some clients who could benefit from good hypnotherapy will not so benefit because they will believe that it did not work for them, when the problem lies not with the technique or themselves, but rather with the hypnotist's lack of psychotherapeutic skill. Good clinical skills are difficult to learn through books. The techniques described in Chapters 3 to 7 are mostly aimed at therapists already trained in the use of clinical hypnosis. If you are not in this category, we strongly recommend that you take some professional workshops, followed by individual or small-group training with a supervisor who is skilled in hypnotherapy.

Hypnotic inductions consists of directing the subject to engage in *detailed focused attention*. It does not seem to matter what the person is focusing on. The focus can range from internal images to external perceptions. It is quite simple as long as you utilize three important principles. First, like traditional forms of Eastern meditation, trance is an experience in focusing and refocusing attention. No one does it perfectly *ever*, especially at the beginning of his or her trance training. The hypnotist must constantly remind patients that they will lose their focus for various reasons (thoughts will come through their minds, the office phone will ring, and so on), so that if they lose focus all they need to do is refocus their attention. Without such a reminder, patients will often tell themselves that they cannot do trance, which will move them from the needed focused attention to an evaluation mode of thinking, thereby causing another negative self-fulfilling prophecy to come true.

The second required principle to utilize for trance inductions is flexibility. Some subjects can focus on anything the hypnotist directs their attention to, while others are more limited in what they will respond to. This is never a problem if you remember that there are no right or wrong ways to do this, only effective versus ineffective ways; no failures, only feedback. For example, suppose after having the subject take a few deep breaths you ask him or her to visualize a chalkboard because you are planning to use a standardized induction involving numbers on that chalkboard. If after a moment it becomes clear that the patient is having trouble with internal visualization, all the hypnotist needs to convey to that patient, through both words and a congruent relaxed attitude, is, "That's okay, no problem, just open your eyes and find a spot on the wall above my shoulder and stare at it, please, while I talk to you." This may seem like a very simple concept, yet too many therapists press what is not working until the patient begins to get the "I am a failure" message and then all kinds of bad things begin to happen to the therapy.

The third induction principle is use of what Bandler and Grinder (1979) call "pacing." Pacing means that the hypnotherapist gets into the patient's world by mirroring him or her in words and rhythm. With patients who are breathing quickly, the therapist should talk more quickly than usual for a while, and then lead them by gradually talking more slowly. Likewise, for patients who from the beginning seem very slowed down, the therapist should slow his or her pace. If we ask patients to focus on their bodies and pay attention to how a given body part is as they inhale and as they exhale, we will say the words "inhale" and "exhale" while the patients are actually doing the same. When we direct subjects to focus their attention if we notice them swallow hard or move an arm we will say, "And as you swallow (or move your arm) you can continue to notice. . . ." The basic idea is to utilize cues from the patient's behavior and then feed back these cues.

By doing this we take what patients will be internally labeling as disruptive, signs that "prove" their lack of ability for trance, and make these behaviors part of the trance induction itself. After a while it seems to many patients that they are doing what we are saying (not vice versa), and it becomes "proof" to them of their cooperation with us.

As we said, the art of hypnotherapy lies in establishing a trusting relationship between the subject and the therapist. By giving the patient permission to drop one focus and then refocus, by maintaining flexibility, and by pacing the patient's rhythm and behaviors with appropriate words, the therapist not only enhances the trance induction, but creates the best environment for productive psychotherapeutic work.

Pacing as an induction principle can include other elements also. For example, if a patient's primary representational system of experiencing is ascertained to be visual, then beginning that patient with a hypnotic induction that involves visualization (for example, staring at a spot or imagining a chalkboard with numbers) might facilitate hypnotic induction at the outset of therapy more than a kinesthetic type of induction such as suggestions that the patient is letting go comfortably in a bathtub full of warm water or a simple arm levitation that would not include visual imagery. A patient who is attending a 12-step recovery program such as Alcoholics Anonymous might be helped to go into trance by imagining going up to the 12th step on a flight of stairs and then stepping out to his or her favorite place; this kind of induction might pace that patient's world that much more and thus facilitate communication, increased empowerment, and change.

What are the therapeutic values of this focused attention trance experience? First, the subject learns to *slow down*. In this fast-paced culture where children grow up in homes where parents watch television, read the newspaper, and talk to them all at the same time, training the mind to slow down and center its attention is in itself helpful. Anxiety is reduced as a consequence of physical changes in the body associated with relaxation. For many patients, anxiety is also reduced as they learn to focus on the present. Most anxiety is anticipatory in nature. When one is fully focused on the present, the future does not exist; therefore no anticipatory responses are elicited. A second value of this focused attention is that the subject learns to concentrate on the experience of the moment. This concentration allows the emergence of details that are often helpful in problem solving. As Sam Keen (1991) has noted, "God lives in the details."

A third therapeutic advantage of a trance experience is that patients learn to suspend the ruminating voice of judgment that usually yammers inside their heads. This judgment is like the self-concept we talked about in the previous chapter. It is problematic even when it is positive and can be devastating when it is critical—as it so often is for our patients. As a person becomes totally aware of and focused on the event at hand, there is less mental "space" for the judgmental voice.

Last, for hypnotherapy, another important aspect of trance is the improved ability of the subject to experience and use visualization. Our existential hypnotherapy uses visualization as an important diagnostic and therapeutic tool (we discuss this topic in Chapter 4).

Even though in Chapter 1 we stated that theoretically we believe all hypnosis is dual hypnosis, belonging to the therapist–patient dialogue, there is a class of experience we label for the patient as self-hypnosis. These types of experiences have important clinical value and will be discussed in some detail in Chapter 6.

Let Go and Travel Light

Man, like a camel, kneels down and lets himself be well-loaded: he loads too many alien grave words and values on himself, and then life seems a desert to him.

—ZARATHUSTRA

I know just what I'd do if I could go back in time somehow, but there's nothing I can do about it now.

—WILLIE NELSON

HOLDING ON TO POWERLESSNESS

Clearly, feeling one's personal power is the ultimate characteristic of the healthy person and therefore the best outcome of psychotherapy. Why, then, is this idea resisted so? Why do behaviorists, the most popular school of psychology in Western culture, believe we are a series of stimulus–response connections, strengthened by reinforcement, rather than free, powerful beings? There are three major reasons for the popularity of stimulus–response or reinforcement theory, each of which has implications for psychotherapy. The last of these reasons has major implications for hypnotherapy.

The first and most obvious reason for the popularity of stimulus–response theory is that if our present behavior is predictable, based on past patterns of reinforcement, then of course we cannot be held responsible for our predicaments. What happens to us, and where we find ourselves, is therefore the fault of the "They"—Heidegger's brilliant self-explana-tory term. "I would be fine if it were not for my parents, my spouse, my school system, my culture," and so on. Responsibility is the child of freedom. Affirming that "I am responsible for my life, the good as well as the bad," is the healthiest of all psychological stances. It is the position that allows for the most growth and change. But it is also a belief that frightens many people in our culture. It is easier to blame the cigarette companies for self-destructive behavior than it is to accept responsibility for the smoking habit and vow to break it once and for all. Preaching the gospel of freedom and responsibility is the job of therapists because the bottom line is that people are really different from worms, pigeons, and rats, and all psychological theories that fail to accept this fundamental truth are flawed. People and animals differ in essential ways: people have a will to power and the ability to change themselves.

A second reason for the success of stimulus–response or reinforcement theory is a widespread fear of not being perfect coupled with a fear of our own pathology. Many psychological theorists have observed that when people get a picture of themselves being at their best, most react with fear and withdraw from that image. Freud (1949) called this the Oceanic complex. Maslow (1971) referred to it as the Joshua complex. The Jungian analyst James Hillman, in his brilliant book *Revisioning Psychology* (1975, p. 55), writes,

> . . . our fear of being what we really are is partly because we fear the psychopathological aspect of individuality. For we are each peculiar; we have symptoms; we fail, and cannot see why we go wrong or even where, despite high hopes and good intentions . . . our insights are impotent, or none come at all. Our feelings disappear in apathy; we worry and also don't care . . . we cannot redeem broken trusts, hopes, loves.

All therapists have the job of helping patients understand that to be perfectly human means to be imperfectly human, to suffer failure as well as success. The most psychologically powerful and healthy people still do not always get what they desire. This, however, can never be an excuse for not trying.

The third issue that explains the popularity of stimulus–

response theory, which in turn blocks the actualization of personal power, is poetically described by Nietzsche in his classic work *Thus Spake Zarathustra* (1954b, p. 25):

> Will that is the name of the liberator and joy bringer; but now learn this too: the Will itself is still a prisoner. Willing liberates; but what is it that puts even the liberator himself in fetters? "It was"—that is the name of the Will's teeth gnashing and most secret melancholy. Powerless against what has been done, he is an angry spectator of the past. The Will cannot will backwards—he cannot break time. . . . "That which was" is the name of the stone he cannot move.
> . . . He wreaks revenge on whatever does not feel wrath and displeasure as he does. Thus the liberated Will took to hurting. This alone is what revenge is. *The Will's ill will against time and its "it was."* (our emphasis)

We have validated Nietzsche's observation in our clinical practice. When patients do good work and begin to get in touch with their personal power, they usually simultaneously get in touch with feelings associated with their past, such as hurt, sadness, fear, or anger. Apparently, the new sense of empowerment helps patients to feel safer and better equipped to deal with these uncomfortable feelings from the past. Their new sense of power also seems to reveal just how powerless these people were or at least felt themselves to be in prior times. As Nietzsche pointed out, anger or rage about the past is often present. Following the anger, the patient experiences massive frustration because even a new-felt sense of empowerment cannot begin to change personal history. That anger and frustration often leads to a psychological aggression that scares patients, often scaring them away from their newfound sense of power and control.

LETTING GO OF THE PAST
AND SELF-CONCEPT

Later in the passage of *Zarathustra* cited above, Nietzsche discusses his belief that in the end, the Will to Power must seek something beyond revenge or even reconciliation. We believe that the "something" is the ability to *let go* of the past. Letting go is moving beyond forgiving or forgetting. It is a deep conscious and unconscious understanding of the epigraph from Willie Nelson at the beginning of this chapter: *"there's nothing I can do about it now."* This needs to be understood as a fact of life, with no particular feeling (happy or sad) associated with it.

The ability to *let go of the past* is such a critical part of learning to be personally powerful that we will devote this first clinical chapter to the use of hypnosis and hypnotherapeutic tasks for this purpose. We use these techniques to some degree with all of our patients.

As we discussed in Chapter 1, letting go means learning to slowly let go of *all* perceptions that people have about themselves; this bundle of perceptions is commonly referred to as "self-concept." We believe that the degree of personal power and self-actualization one achieves directly correlates with one's ability to let go of labels. Living beings are transitory. All being is becoming. Try to grasp something and the act of grasping itself changes it. As the Buddha pointed out, all suffering comes from clinging. Hermann Hesse shows us in his classic novel *Siddhartha* that letting go of self-definition even means letting go of those classifications that on the surface seem positive. Hesse (1951, p. 33) said that when Siddhartha found he was no longer a Brahmin of high standing, no longer a nobleman, no ascetic belonging to the Samanas, he was nothing but Siddhartha, he felt more alone than any hermit. He was overwhelmed by a feeling of icy despair, but *he was more firmly himself than ever* (our emphasis) and on the road to true enlightenment.

We will begin this discussion by explaining the use of hypnotic trance as a framework that helps patients to let go of the past and other dysfunctional realities as they generate new healthier realities for themselves.

HYPNOTIC TECHNIQUES FOR LETTING GO

Milton Erickson was the first practitioner to conceive of hypnotic trance, in and of itself, as an experience that reorganizes one's realities. Erickson (1980, Vol. 4, p. 38) states, "The induction and maintenance of a trance serve to provide a special psychological state in which the patient can reassociate and reorganize his inner psychological complexities and utilize his own capacities in a manner in accord with his own experiential life." This view contrasts with traditional views of hypnosis that employ trance to condition or program the patient by use of suggestions. Erickson sees trance as the fertile ground for healthy new experience and new realities self-generated by the patient, based on his or her own history, and entailing a letting go of unhealthy past realities. The hypnotist does not direct the patient to adopt realities the hypnotist suggests; no, the hypnotist merely facilitates the patient's own search for realities that make sense for him or her. Viewing trance in this way and explaining this view to patients is more empowering: the patient will start to feel better as soon as he or she realizes that new realities arise from and are the work of the patient, not the hypnotist. All patients need to learn that perception is determined by the combination of personal history and present motivation. They also need to learn that there is always another way to look at anything. In fact, most relationship problems occur because two people have different perceptions of the same thing.

To illustrate our views about the value of trance and our method of using trance, we will not offer a sample of the typical hypnotic dialogue we use early in the therapy of a patient. Ordinarily, words such as these would be spoken during a first session of formal hypnosis with a patient, just after the patient enters a trance state of experience.

"John, everyone who walks into this office comes in with his own realities and perceptions about his life—his past, present, and future—and about his world that that person is reacting to as if these are truths. However, you might agree with me that there are few truths in this universe, and many would argue that there are no truths, John— just an infinite array of realities available to us. For example, any million men living your life would have a million different perceptions or evaluations about it, different in at least some ways. No doubt, there would be those who would think that your life is much more positive than how you have been experiencing it, and there would be those that would generally agree with you in your perceptions, and there would be those who would evaluate your life as much crummier than you. The point is, where is the truth in all this? It's nice to tell you, John, that with trance experiencing, there is a subtle suspension of the ordinary realities, perceptions, and frameworks that you have been walking around with and reacting to as truths. A bridge is generated to the unconscious mind—trance is that bridge—and there in your unconscious, John, safely stored there, is the experiences of your entire life. That is a tremendous resource for you. And with trance experiencing this resource is tapped into, and automatically new realities are created for you to experience. New ways to see, think, hear, and feel about your life that are healthier for you. These new realities that you will be experiencing are no more truthful than the other ones that have gotten in the way; they are just healthier and more comfortable, John. Every time we do hypnosis or you do self-hypnosis, this process of new realities, which will be your new truths, is being synthesized for you."

For all our patients, we frame hypnotic trance as a letting-go experience. We suggest to patients that just by experiencing the trance state, old unhealthy patterns or realities will disappear and be replaced by more comfortable, healthier patterns and realities. This suggestion by itself often frees the patient, gives him or her "permission" or a good reason, to experience his or her world differently.

UNBLOCKING AND RESOLVING PAST EXPERIENCE BY MEANS OF TRANCE

Hypnosis is widely used to unblock traumatically dissociated amnesiac memories. The negative energy associated with these memories often gets in the way of healthier functioning. However, because of the traumatic amnesia involved, a patient may not even know that current symptoms are associated with past trauma or, to use language consistent with our discussion, that the past has not been let go of. For example, sexual problems may be associated with long-forgotten child sexual abuse trauma.

Regression techniques are well documented and are often helpful, even though the accuracy of data obtained "from the past" is a controversial issue (Scheflin & Shapiro, 1989). Hypnotic regression could be employed simply by suggesting that the patient go back in memory and remember a trauma related to current symptoms. Of course, the clinician should be prepared to deal with the possibility of catharsis or abreaction stimulated by painful affect.

The use of the image of the patient's "inner child" or "child within" and related "reparenting" strategies are becoming increasingly popular (see Bradshaw, 1990; Capacchione, 1991; King, Golden, King, & Citrenbaum, 1989; Whitfield, 1987). These techniques are useful as a vehicle for regression to and exploration of the past and any trauma that may have occurred then, as well as for working through wounds associated with the past. These techniques can be used successfully to encourage letting go. As is the case when using any kind of imagery, "inner child" and "reparenting" frameworks are most powerful when the patient is experiencing hypnotic trance. To the best of our knowledge, the first person to employ such strategies was Milton Erickson, as he reveals while discussing the case of the February Man (Erickson & Rossi, 1979, chap. 10). Others who use such concepts include Hugh Missildine, who wrote the important book *Your Inner Child of the Past* (1982), Eric Berne (1961) and other practitioners of transactional analysis, and Alice Miller (1984).

Here is a transcript of a typical communication that we might use with a hypnotized patient in order to introduce her to her "inner child" and to begin associated work within that framework:

"Mary, would you imagine that you are walking on a path that stretches out before you. Please imagine that you can see what's on the path, hear any sound associated with walking on the path, and that you can feel the dirt beneath your feet. Imagine the path stretches out before you. Please imagine that, up in the distance, you can begin to see the image of a little person who is slowly walking toward you. Please imagine that now you can see that this little person is a little girl. Would you imagine now that you can see as this little girl gets closer to you, that she looks just like you, Mary, when you were a little girl. Mary, this is your inner child or the child within you. This little girl has always been living there in your mind, your heart, your tummy, or other places, and she is the inner part of you who is so very much responsible for your sensitivities, your feeling, and other bodily stuff. Imagine that the two of you are approaching each other and nod your head, please, when she is right there in front of you. [Patient nods her head. At this point, we may ask the patient to tell us about how old this child looks, what the child is wearing, and whether the child has a nickname or a name other than what the patient's current name is.] If it's okay with you, Mary, you can ask that little girl if she would like a hug and then you can imagine giving her a nice big hug. Now you can spend some moments with her and let her know that you want to help her out. You can also let her know that you know for sure that she survives it all, since you're living proof of that; and that she has you now, with all of your experiences and power, to help her. There may be some things that you want to say to her that you know she could use hearing, Mary. For example, you could tell her that she is a lovable, valuable child and that she's okay just the way she is."

At this point, the patient can be led into helping out this child through reparenting nurturing strategies, and rendering positive communication to the child. The patient can take the child for a walk and have fun with the child. The patient can even be led into imagining meeting healthy parental figures on the path that can help out with reparenting the child. These images can be based on the patient's own parents, who are behaving in a positive healthy way, or on any people that the patient would like to imagine as parents.

Past trauma can be dealt with by allowing the patient to see the image of the inner child enduring that trauma. This technique often stimulates cartharsis of the painful affect that is associated with that trauma. The patient can be encouraged to imagine "rescuing" the "inner child" by imagining the beginning of the traumatic scenario and then jumping in and warding off the abuse or some other similar strategy, thereby creating a new scenario or, conceivably, a new history, for the patient (Quigley, 1989). Keep in mind that some traumatized patients may require "distance" when first remembering and dealing with traumatic past events. Dissociative strategies, for example, suggesting to patients that they imagine themselves in a theater viewing a movie of the episode, often prove helpful. Suggesting to the patient that he or she is holding a control panel that controls the speed, clarity, or size of the images in the movie can provide increased safety. These techniques allow the patient to view the past with the full knowledge and power of an adult. Trauma does not need to be reexperienced as trauma for therapy to be effective!

We consider the "inner child" to be a kind of metaphor. In Chapter 7 we will discuss the use of metaphors to alter the existential reality of patients. In a more intelligent world we would not have to explain that, for us, the "inner child" is a useful image, not a reality. Today, however, there are so many "new age" writers who present the "inner child" as an entity in itself, a kind of being within the being, that we want to dissociate ourselves from this belief while not throwing out the baby with the bath water. This metaphor of the "inner child" seems to pace the reality of many clients and is therefore often therapeutically useful.

GESTALT THERAPY TECHNIQUES

In terms of gestalt therapy, patients hold on to the past, and thus feel anxious, guilty, or depressed, when they have not "completed" an experience or formed the gestalt associated with that part of their past. Usually, this means that a person has not fully expressed himself or herself in some necessary manner, and therefore is stuck with a negative feeling that gets in the way of feeling personal power in his or her current life. Gestalt techniques, therefore, consist of strategies to help people complete their experiences in order to "let go" of something they have been holding onto, such as anger, hurt, guilt, or fear. To use gestalt terms, the patient is helped to bring into the "foreground" what has been in the "background." If someone is feeling anxious or depressed, but does not know why—a common enough experience—then a gestalt therapist assumes that the patient is harboring a feeling or experience that has not been fully felt or experienced, usually because the feeling or experience was too threatening to work through when it originated. Gestalt techniques consist of moving this experience out of the dark into the person's awareness, or consciousness. The background must become foreground, must be viewed, examined, experienced honestly, to be able to let it go. To a gestalt therapist a person must first *be* with an experience in order to let it go. To a gestalt therapist, the only way out of anxiety or discomfort is through it. Gestalt techniques consist of awareness exercises and expressive techniques to take care of unfinished business.

Gestalt therapy strategies always include hypnotic experiences, even though writers with a gestalt therapy framework usually do not label hypnosis as hypnosis. As we understand these gestalt techniques, they require a focused attention that produces a natural trance experience. We have noticed that the therapeutic value of gestalt-type techniques seems to increase when we label these strategies "hypnosis" for our patients and begin use of these techniques *after* a formal trance induction. We believe that use of the hypnotic label and a formal trance induction enhances the overall process by utilizing the placebo effect of hypnosis we discussed earlier. For example, such use may provide some patients the permission they need to "talk to an empty chair" (a technique discusswed later in this chapter).

We will discuss four of the gestalt techniques we have found to be particularly useful in existential hypnotherapy.

Bodily or Feeling Awareness and Augmentation

Have the patient close his or her eyes and attend to the body, reporting any tightness, tension, or discomfort. At the report of any experience like this—for example, "My throat feels tight"—the therapist should instruct the patient to attend to the experience and amplify this experience to increase awareness by the patient. When the patient amplifies this negative experience, instead of constraining or suppressing it (the patient's presumed habitual pattern), and allows himself or herself to have the experience, very often the experience or feeling is completed. Having completed the experience, the patient is able to let it go. In the example just described, the patient might spontaneously start to cry, or get angry, or might even become aware of other associations attached to the feeling; thus hurt or anger associated with a particular past event or a significant person in the patient's life might be called up and experienced in association with the throat tightening the patient is experiencing.

A variation of this gestalt technique of amplifying a bodily experience or feeling is to suggest to the patient that he or she use his or her imagination to *become* the experience or the part of the body upon which attention is being focused. For example, the therapist may point out to a patient that his hand had just closed into a fist when he was talking about his mother. The therapist might then request the patient to imagine becoming that fist and talk about itself or what it feels like doing. Becoming the experience or feeling or part of the body can increase the patient's awareness of a suppressed or repressed or "uncompleted" feeling or experience so that the feeling can be addressed and dealt with. For example, one patient, upon request by her therapist, imagined becoming her hand and quite spontaneously spoke of wanting to hit her mother right in the gut. When the "fist" or the patient imagined doing this, then the patient's hand was able to relax; that is, the feeling of anger was completed so that it could be dismissed, be let go.

The "Empty Chair" Technique

This classical and popular gestalt technique consists of placing a chair in front of the patient, who then imagines a person with whom he or she has "unfinished business." One patient who was enraged at his deceased father was asked by the therapist to imagine his father in the empty chair and then the patient, with the therapist's support, said what he had long needed to say to his father and truly expressed himself.

Gestalt theory (Perls, Hefferline, & Goodman, 1951; Perls, 1969) states that when patients become aware of feelings or experience and attend to these feelings and express themselves, letting go of the experience occurs automatically. However, we feel that it is still important to *communicate* to the patient the importance of letting go. We would say something like this: "Since you have been doing this good work and are taking care of this business, John, now you can let go of your anger and feel more comfortable and powerful."

"Here and Now" Awareness Exercises

Gestalt therapists value full experiencing of the moment "in the here and now" in order to achieve completion, and then a moving on to the next experience from one moment to moment. Numerous gestalt exercises reinforce full experiencing in the here and now. All of these exercises are quite hypnotic; in fact, each can be considered a hypnotic induction. Here is an example of a strategy that is often helpful for patients. Ask the patient to state out loud, "Here and now I am aware of . . . ," and then to finish this statement with whatever the patient is aware of at that moment. The phrase must then be repeated and completed again with whatever the patient's experience is at that particular moment, and then again, and again. We recommend that the therapist model use of this technique for the patient. We also recommend utilizing as many sensory modalities as possible: for example, "Here and now I am aware of breathing out. Here and now I am aware of seeing the smile on your face. Here and now I am aware of feeling the leather of the armrest below my hands. Here and now I am aware of hearing the phone ring in the office next door," and so on. Regular use of this strategy by a patient promotes here and now experiencing, in contrast to living in the past or already being in the future.

Mock Funerals

This rather dramatic therapeutic technique gives the patient the opportunity to "bury" something or someone that the patient has been holding onto, something or someone that is getting in the way of a more fulfilling and productive life. Patients can "bury" a destructive habit such as cigarette smoking or alcoholism, an old relationship, a person who has literally died but is still alive within that patient, or just about anything.

Mock funerals utilize the power of rituals, a part of the socialization of all of us, to help us make a transition, to help us to let go of the past and move on. The more ritualized or "real" a therapeutic funeral is, the more power it has in helping a patient to let go of something that is not needed anymore. We have directed mock funerals in a therapeutic group situation in which everyone in the group became part of the funeral procession and helped to bury a mock casket containing objects symbolic of what the patients were letting go of. We have also used therapeutic funerals in one-to-one therapy situations. We help the patient to "buy into" a funeral in order to bury, and therefore to let go of, something the patient needs to dispose of—for example, feelings of hurt and anger caused by an old girlfriend. We direct that patient to come to his next session dressed appropriately for a funeral, and to bring along objects associated with the old girlfriend—perhaps old love letters or photographs—that will be buried. We also ask him to bring a eulogy focused upon letting go of the feelings for this person from the past. We ask the patient's consent to allow our secretary (known to the patient from his frequent sessions) to be present as a witness at the funeral. At the patient's next therapy appointment a cardboard box draped in black is set up at the front of the therapy room on a table surrounded by candles, and the therapist and secretary, dressed in black, are already waiting in chairs facing this "coffin." During the "funeral" the patient reads his eulogy and the therapist speaks some appropriate words. Then the patient is directed to bury the "coffin." This latter directive usually involves the patient digging a "grave." After this kind of work, which some therapists like Jay Haley (1984) might call "ordeal therapy," the patient is even more invested in the whole process of letting go of the feelings that were buried. We even direct some patients return to the "grave" daily for a designated period of time to "mourn." Therapists who have never engaged in techniques of this dramatic nature would be quite surprised at how seriously most patients will take the whole procedure, especially if it is proposed in a rather serious way by the therapist, and at how powerful such strategies can be in helping a patient to let go of the past.

HYPNOTIC MEDITATION

We often use a successful technique that combines hypnotic suggestion with a classic meditation experience, following one's breath. This technique is particularly effective when the patient needs to learn to let go of a recurring thought or feeling such as anger or anxiety. During a patient's trance we make the hypnotic suggestion that when she stops whatever she is doing for just a moment and follows her breath in and out three times, then she will feel more centered and be able to "let go" of anger (or whatever). We direct the patient to follow that breath all the way down to the pit of the stomach and then up again and out, while saying to herself, "Breath in, breath out" three times. What we do here is set up a classic "when–then" message (which is the essence of hypnotic suggestion). We tell the patient that *when* she follows the breath in this way, *then* she will let go of the unwanted feeling. If we have established therapeutic credibility with the patient, the technique works because the patient believes us when we tell her it will work.

To increase the effectiveness of this technique we have patients imagine a common problematic situation while in trance. For example, one patient came to therapy because she regularly raged at other people. During a session she was directed to imagine she was in her kitchen and her teenage daughter entered, engaging in the kind of behavior that usually caused the patient to experience explosive rage. The patient was then told to stop all her behavioral responses for just a moment and to focus on her breath. She was then asked to imagine how to respond to her daughter in an appropriate way, a way that allowed her to feel in control. Such suggestions combined with "practice" in an office context seem to have a therapeutic effect for a significant percentage of our patient population.

EMBEDDED SUGGESTIONS

This communication strategy, also known as *analogue marking*, was pioneered by Milton Erickson (Erickson, 1966; Erickson & Rossi, 1976a), who called it the *interspersal technique*, and popularized by John Grinder and Richard Bandler (Grinder & Bandler, 1981). An embedded suggestion is a form of communication that is not apparent to the patient's conscious perception or mind, but it does register in the patient's unconscious mind. These suggestions can be given to the patient within the context of formal trance, but they can also be communicated easily during any clinical communication ("little-*h* hypnosis").

As we discussed in previous works (King et al., 1983; Citrenbaum et al., 1985), embedded suggestions bypass conscious analysis and the resistance that can interfere with change. Such techniques, even when rendered outside a context that includes a formal hypnotic induction, are directed to the right brain hemisphere, the "seat of the unconscious." Here they are capable of being quite influential. Numerous studies (see Springer & Deutsch, 1981) have documented the power of communication directed to the right side of the brain, as well as people's lack of conscious awareness of such influence.

A good deal of research (Smith, Chu, & Edmonston, 1977; Diamond & Beaumont, 1974; Kinsbourne & Smith, 1974) has concluded that when the dominant cerebral hemisphere of the brain is focused on some task, the other hemisphere is free to receive and deal with other information. Erickson and Rossi (1979, p. 261) stated that "this may be the neuropsychological basis of [Erickson's] practice of interspersing suggestions in the symbolic language of the unconscious."

Subtly increasing the volume of one's voice when delivering the embedded suggestion is the easiest way to use this technique in most clinical situations. Allowing a slight pause before and after such suggestions (indicated by italics preceded and followed by a dash [—] in our examples) and attaching the patient's name to them can empower embedded suggestions even more. We might say, for example, "Learning from the past can be helpful, but otherwise it's healthy to—*let go of the past, Tom*—move on."

The kinesthetic sense can also be used to deliver embedded suggestions; for example, the clinician can lean over and put a hand on the patient's hand, arm, or shoulder while communicating an embedded suggestion. This act of touching helps to highlight that communication to the unconscious.

A visual embedded suggestion, which can only be used when the patient's eyes are open and the patient is watching the clinician, can also be utilized. The clinician can lift his or her arms in a bracketing type of gesture when the key words comprising the suggestion are communicated. Advertising and other announcements commonly use visual embedded suggestions by highlighting the embedded suggestion through use of a bolder typeface, italics, or other visual means. To illustrate further, we, the authors, hope that you, the reader, will *let go* of ineffective communication strategies, but we know that this will occur only when *you are ready to*.

Often we tell stories or use metaphors to convey specific therapeutic messages. We will discuss this practice in detail in Chapter 7; here we will offer just a brief description. When we begin formal trance work, we usually tell one or two stories strictly for the purpose of being able to repeat, as an embedded suggestion, a "let go" message. These messages serve a dual purpose when given as part of the patter during the trance induction. First, the patient gets the message to "let go" of ordinary experience and go into trance; second, these messages also serve as suggestions to "let go" of symptoms. Here is an example of the kinds of stories we tell for the purpose of delivering embedded messages about letting go:

"I've been lucky enough to travel around this country teaching hypnosis to professionals. Wherever I go the participants have a copy of my latest couple of books. One of these books has a picture of a roller coaster on the front cover and people ask what that has to do with trance or helping people like you with their problems. I tell them that the secret of going into trance, and the secret of helping people like you with these kinds of problems, and the secret of riding a roller coaster are all the same thing—it's the task of learning when to hold on and learning when to—*let go, Fred*. I have a 17-year-old daughter who, when she was very young, just 9 or 10, already knew the secret so she could safely ride any roller coaster in the world. She knew that when the roller coaster was steaming down the hill and around the bend she had to hold on tight because that's what's safe and comfortable for someone her size and age. But even at an early age she noticed that there were people in life who always held on and those people ended up with sore hands or stiff elbows, pains in the back, pains in the neck, or even headaches. She knew, as do you, there were times when the roller coaster was going up the first hill and you could literally hear the clanking of the chain pulling it up, that's the time you could sit back and—*let go, Fred*—or when the roller coaster was near the top of the first hill and you could enjoy the view of whatever park you were in, that's the time that you could just—*let go, Fred*—because both your conscious mind and what I call your unconscious mind—my daughter just jokingly calls it her woman's intuition—will let you know when to hold on again."

After telling that story we continue on with the hypnotic session and doing whatever we are about to do. We never consciously discuss this story. Obviously, the only reason to tell it is to repeat "*let go*"as often as possible. One of the things that never ceases to amaze us is that about 25% of our patients, within 2 weeks, come back in and say, "You know, [Dr. King or Dr. Citrenbaum], this past week I was walking around the shopping mall and I began to get those old panic attacks like I used to have and then there was a little voice inside my head that said, 'Why don't you just let go' and I was able to take a deep breath and do that. I wonder why that happened?" Of course, we just smile. It is amazing how few of our patients remember that we even told the roller coaster story or made any similar kind of suggestion to them. This is the ultimate form of therapeutic empowerment because the patient gets all the credit for the change: they do not even remember we had anything to do with it.

A case example provides a picture of how we use stories early in our therapeutic work, while the patient is learning to experience trance. John had an avid interest in airplanes and in flying. He had come to therapy suffering from high blood pressure and other stress-related symptoms. Generally, John seemed to take life much too seriously. He was an adult child of an alcoholic and always needed to be perfect in everything he did. A therapeutic story we used in treating him demonstrates how we utilize the patient's own interests and personality in developing our metaphors. Again, we were trying to communicate the single but effective message, "Let go."

"You know, John, one thing that you and I and all my friends and all your friends have in common is that we all want to be in control. That's natural enough. Often times each of us makes the mistake of thinking that being in control means holding on tight when often the opposite is true. Now and then we each need to relearn this lesson. I needed to relearn it myself about 7 years ago. I was learning how to fly single-engine planes and, as you may or may not know, flying planes is actually quite easy, but landing one is difficult. In fact, you've probably heard the old saying that anyone can fly a plane, but it takes a pilot to land one. Well, you can understand that I always wanted my landings to be perfect, so I used to hold the wheel called an aileron tight and my instructor was always shouting to me to—*let go, let go*—but I wanted to be in control and so I held on tight. I learned to fly safely enough so I could fly by myself and one day I was practicing my landings, just doing touch-and-goes around the airport, when I made a particularly bad landing—I just bounced down the runway like a kangaroo. I was so disgusted with myself that the next time around doing the downwind leg I just heard my instructor's voice in the back of my mind shouting to me—*let go, let go, John*—that's what he said. I thought what did I have to lose? So, I took a deep breath and—*let go*—totally with one hand. The other hand I held gently as I would a car with power steering that I was comfortable with, and wouldn't you know, when I learned to—*let go*—I had so much more control I was able to land the plane perfectly, right on the numbers as we call it. So that was another lesson that I had learned about holding on and letting go and being in control."

Once again all the "let go's," usually with the patient's name attached, are said with a slight tonal shift (a rise or deepening of the voice) and a slight pause before and after. These practices help to embed the "let go" phrase in the unconscious.

IMAGERY

As we will discuss in detail in Chapter 4, imagery is the language of the unconscious. Thus images can be particularly powerful in helping people to let go of the past. Merely telling a patient to "let go" of something or someone from the past is not an effective therapy; he or she has heard that advice many times before from family and friends—too many times for it to have much meaning. But helping a patient to *experience* or to *imagine* letting go is quite different and potentially more productive.

One method of using imagery to help a person to let go of the past is to simply ask the patient to imagine or visualize in some symbolic way what his or her feeling associated with the past looks like and then to utilize that imagery in a therapeutic way. For example, one patient who constantly complained of feeling tense and weighted down because of feelings for his ex-wife was asked to close his eyes and to imagine what this experience within himself looked like. He described the feeling of his ex-wife as a "big, grey boulder blocking my way." When the therapist asked the patient what would help to get rid of this boulder, the patient generated an image of workers with jackhammers coming along to break the boulder up into smaller pieces that could be hauled away. The patient was then directed to spend 3 or 4 minutes every day closing his eyes and imagining these workers demolishing the boulder. When the patient returned 1 week later he reported feeling better and indicated that he had been able to start asking other women out on dates.

Here is an imagining exercise involving the patient's "excess baggage" that we regularly use, often as a "self-hypnosis" assignment. The patient, with eyes closed, is asked to imagine going to the "attic" of his or her mind and to imagine finding his or her "excess baggage," and then to dispose of that excess baggage from the past. The therapist can use this image of excess baggage in a variety of ways. Here is one specific example of the use of this image in the form of a verbatim transcript of a therapeutic directive given to one patient:

"Jim, this week when you are in trance while doing self-hypnosis I would like you to imagine that you go up to the attic of your mind and that you go into your attic and that you find your excess baggage. Jim, this is stuff that you've been carrying around with you from the past and that's been weighing you down and using up your energy needlessly and that you don't need to have with you anymore. This is stuff that may have been helpful to you at some other time, but now it's just getting in the way. Unfortunately, it's quite common to keep holding onto things like this, Jim. All I want you to do is find this excess baggage and take a look at the containers and see what they look like, Jim. See how big or small they are, the size and shapes of these containers and maybe even what kind of material they are made out of—but you don't even have to bother with the contents. You may have some guesses as to what's inside these bags and that's just your unconscious mind, and only your unconscious will know for sure. Whatever excess baggage you find in the attic of your mind, I'd like you to imagine bringing out of the attic and having those bags here with you next time, Jim, for the opportunity to *let them go.*"

When the patient comes in for his next session we will then let him imagine that he "drops off" or "lets go" of his excess baggage in the office or somewhere else. Patients can be asked to bring in excess baggage from the "basement" of their mind also.

Here is an example of the hypnotic dialogue that might be used to help a patient let go of excess baggage:

"Jim, you indicated before going into trance that you did bring in excess baggage as I had asked you to, and now I want to give you the opportunity to help yourself out by being able to—*let go of that baggage, Jim.* Please take a few moments now, and imagine that you gather up your excess baggage and that you then just put that stuff down here on the floor. If you need more room you can use the hallway outside. Just make sure that you leave a path for people to walk by. Once in a while, Jim, someone will become aware that they just can't let go of one or two

Let Go and Travel Light

pieces of excess baggage. That usually means that your unconscious doesn't feel quite safe enough to let go of those bags just yet, Jim. So it's okay, if this is the case with you, to take one or two pieces of excess baggage back home with you until you are ready to—*let go of that baggage also, Jim.* If you are still coming here, you can do it anytime you are here in my office, but you can always imagine letting go of it by yourself too. I know you're a conscientious person, Jim, but you don't have to worry about polluting my space by putting your excess baggage down here. That's because I have a nice agreement with the maintenance people here in this building that they will dispose of any excess baggage that my patients leave here. You'll be happy that you are letting go of this stuff that you don't need anymore, Jim, and one of these days, sooner or later, you'll be aware that you're getting around more lightly and freely. Please nod your head to let me know after you have dropped off your excess baggage."

Another technique we like to employ involves the use of "past and future clocks." One of us (King) has two clocks in his office, one set for 11 hours in the past and the other for 14 hours in the future. The image of these clocks can be utilized to help patients become healthier. Here is an example of suggestions given to a patient named Mary:

"Mary, a friend of mine in Pittsburgh has two clocks on the walls in his office and he and his patients sit right between those clocks. One of those clocks is set for a time in the western Pacific, where it is still yesterday. The clock on the other side of the room is set for a time in England where it is already tomorrow. My friend tells patients that those clocks are there to remind you and others to *live in the present and the here and now, Mary.* He tells them that, unfortunately, too many people are stealing from their experience in the present by still living in the past. These are people who are still resenting someone or something in the past, or who still feel hurt or guilty about the past.

Other people are already looking at what time it is tomorrow, Mary, and preoccupied with the future, and that steals from present moments also. These people are always planning for the future or feel real anxious about it, and they never are really experiencing the comfortable moments that they have now. Some learning from the past and some planning for the future is quite helpful, but otherwise it's so important to *experience your moments now as fully as you can, Mary*. Just remember that every day you get up is today."

These kinds of suggestions can be given to patients in or out of formal trance. The reader can use his or her own creativity to modify the use of such suggestions accordingly. The purpose of the "clocks" exercise is to help the patient let go of obsessing about the past or future. In and of itself, a image like this will not cure a disorder; but each image is a weapon in the battle for recovery.

"LETTING GO" STORIES

We wanted to end this chapter with two of our favorite "letting go" stories. The first concerns two monks:

"Two monks were walking from the town to the temple, a 3-day walk which they did in silence. On the morning of the third day they came across a beautiful woman in a silk kimono standing to one side of a mud puddle. One of the monks picked the woman up and carried her over the mud puddle and put her down. The monks continued to walk in silence and when they got to the foot of the temple, some hours away, the other monk turned and said to him, 'I can't help but say this, but as monks we are not supposed to touch women; it's dangerous.' The other monk turned to him and said, 'I put her down back at the mud puddle half a day ago. Are you still carrying her around with you?'"

The second "letting go" story is a variation of a beautiful and often told Sufi teaching tale:

"Once upon a time there was a stream that flowed down a mountain until it touched the land. Then the stream set out on its journey. Mile after mile, day after day, that stream flowed onward. Sometimes there was a barrier in the path of the stream, but the stream managed to get beyond whatever obstacle lay before it. Then, finally, the stream reached the desert; but as quickly as it flowed into the desert, just as quickly it was absorbed by the desert sand. That stream had traveled a long way over a long period of time, so in the same way it just flowed onward. But just as quickly, it was absorbed by the sand. Then a whisper emerged from the sand. The sand said, 'The wind travels across the desert, so can the stream.' The stream answered, 'Yes, but the wind can fly, a stream can't fly.' 'You can *let yourself go* to the wind,' the sand whispered, 'and it will take you in its arms and carry you across the desert to the other side.' Then the stream felt afraid. It had never experienced anything of that nature, and the stream was afraid to *let go*, for it feared losing its very identity and perhaps never regaining it again. 'Listen,' the sand whispered. 'You are going to change now one way or the other. Whether you *let go* to the wind, or stay right here and continue to try to flow through the sand, you will change. If you *let go* to the wind, it's your essence, your very essence, that the wind will gently take you in its arms and carry you to the other side; and there you will be you again, but changed. If you continue to try to flow into the sand, then the sand will just absorb you and, at most, you will become a quagmire. In either case, you will change,' said the sand. 'The choice is yours.' The stream still felt afraid, but somehow the stream was able to *tap into the courage needed*, and it was able to *let go* to the wind. The wind gently absorbed the very essence of the stream and carried it for many miles and many days across the vast desert to the other side. And when the wind touched the roof of a mountain there, the gentle rain fell; and soon that stream flowed again, essentially itself, but changed too, having learned to trust its true identity even more. The stream flowed down that mountain until it touched the land and then continued on its way. And maybe this is why it's sometimes said that the journey of the stream of life is often whispered by the desert sand."

CHAPTER 4

The Will to Power

In Chapter 1 we stated that from an existential perspective the desired outcome of all psychotherapy is for the patient to experience a sense of personal empowerment. All our hypnotherapy techniques, directly or indirectly, work toward that end. The reader may note that much of our work seems aimed at behavioral changes. Indeed, we believe the fastest way to change feelings about oneself is to change selected behaviors. It is not specific behavioral change, however, that is the measure of successful psychotherapy; the real measure is the experience of "being able to do it." Hypnotherapy can be a particularly effective treatment modality, for it can help patients who initially experience themselves as powerless to learn to experience their personal power.

Existential thinkers do not believe the world (or people) can be properly understood by using linear cause-and-effect thinking. That kind of thinking results from a narrow vision. It is like looking through a picket fence and watching a herd of animals pass by. For each animal, the head precedes the tail. If one stayed long enough at this picket fence one would probably feel very comfortable with the theory that the head caused the tail. Our history is our story and, as Sam Keen (Keen & Fox, 1973) has pointed out, each of us needs to tell our story. This is one of the values of psychotherapy. It does not follow, however, that the history that is our story need be our cause.

Most popular psychology today, as evidenced by the self-help books, the television and radio talk shows, and unfortunately even a lot of professional psychology, promotes the idea that we are caused by—and therefore victims of—our childhood. Too many people today take the unhealthy way and say, "I can't help it, my inner child was starved for affection and made me do it." This psychological concept does bring forth some compassion for those who may have had a rougher childhood than some of us luckier ones. But the negative side effect of this compassion is that large numbers of people are being encouraged to embrace a passive, victim role and are allowed by the "They" to avoid taking personal responsibility for their lives.

Hillman and Ventura (1992) suggest that today's psychology is again emphasizing a looking backward to what Jung called the "child archetype." The child archetype by its nature is both apolitical and disempowered. They argue that this is a disaster at the political level because democracy depends on active citizens, not on adult children. We can add to their thought that personal growth, the kind of growth that good psychotherapy should promote, also requires active, responsible adults, not children. As Father Leo Booth (1992) put it, "Recovery requires that you see yourself not just as a child of God, but as a *powerful* child of God." Therapists who use today's jargon need to understand the importance of patients viewing themselves, for example, not as "adult children of alcoholics" but as "*powerful* adult children of alcoholics."

It is very easy for therapists to get lost in their kindness and not be aware of the damage they cause by promoting the long-term infantilization of the recipient of that kindness. We recently viewed a network television show about pornography and whether it is a form of sexual harassment. A panel of experts was shown a sequence from a pornographic movie in which a young woman in underwear is surrounded by a group of fraternity boys who eye and touch her. The panel members, all seemingly displaying great compassion for the woman, agreed that she was the victim of sexual harassment. Moreover, panel members argued that even if she *seemingly* chose to do what she was doing, this was so only because of economic harassment. (It used to be called "work" when you took your body someplace it often did not want to go because the boss had money you needed.) From our existential frame-work these "caring" professionals did more than the boys in the porn film to put down the woman. None of them could conceive of the possibility that she may have freely chosen to work one night on her back rather than 40 hours on her feet at Sears to earn the same pay. No one allowed her the dignity of being responsible for her choice.

If the woman in this movie were to appear in our office because she was questioning her life and as a consequence suffering from mild anxiety and depression, we would see it as disruptive to the therapy process if we showed our empathy for her suffering by in any way supporting the view of her as a victim. There are other ways to show caring. This patient must learn to accept the existential truth that while there were influences in her life that helped to "shape" her, *she* herself had decided how to respond to each influence, and therefore she herself was the most influential "shaper." Although existential hypnotherapy is much more than just changing the patient's perceptions, the patient must come to understand the relationship between the self and the lived world (*Lebenswelt*) differently. This woman needs the therapist's help to own the choices that are her life. She needs to know that all her choices had payoffs and that they are not random or crazy, but they also had penalties—that is why she needs therapy. Alternative choices will also have their mix of payoffs and penalties; rarely are choices black or white —indeed, it is the grey that produces the anxiety of the unknown. In the end, this woman may keep doing the same things but arrive at a different understanding about herself and what she does. Her specific choices should be of no consequence to the therapist or to the "experts" on television. Therapy can be judged successful only if this patient leaves feeling empowered.

A variety of hypnotherapy techniques are usually needed to help a patient overcome years of socialization (we usually call this "early childhood hypnosis") that encourage him or her to believe that he or she is a victim of circumstance. Many people prefer the comfort of lack of responsibility. Certainly, some people are victims of other people's evil or mental illness, or of circumstances. Victims of child abuse, rape, criminal assaults, and the like, *are* victims. However, each of these individual victims will respond differently to the misfortune that befalls him or her. One person will recover from an assault whereas another will stay a "victim" for life. Adults are responsible for their response to any event in their lives. It takes a sense of empowerment to recover. It is still *they* who will feel miserable until *they* make some changes. The rest of this chapter will discuss hypnotherapy techniques that are helpful in working with patients on issues concerning such personal power.

For most patients, during the first or second visit, we find some excuse to point to a picture of Milton Erickson that hangs in the office. We say,

> "That is a picture of Dr. Erickson, one of my teachers. Years ago he told me a very interesting story. Right after Pearl Harbor he was a physician for the New York City Draft Board and at that time, of course, men were lined up to enlist. Dr. Erickson told us that one day a man with one arm tried to join the army. After a few minutes Erickson wrote down the words 'Rejected, cripple' and the medical residents following him around all gave their nodding approval. One week later another man walked in who was also missing an arm. Dr. Erickson said he sensed there was something different about this man. He asked the one-armed man to tie his shoe. He was able to do this with one hand. Erickson gave him a variety of other tests, finally asking, 'Is there any reason you shouldn't be in the army?' The man answered, 'Only because I can't salute with the right hand.'"

The point of this story is that being born in a certain way (including in a particular family) does not in itself make one a cripple. Only a person can do that to himself or herself!

Chapter 7 will discuss the reasons for using stories and metaphors in existential hypnotherapy. Many of these metaphors have personal empowerment as their therapeutic aim. We have included two such stories in this chapter, the story about the one-armed man and the one below. The first we tell to almost every patient near the beginning of therapy and the one below is the story we tell at or near termination. The latter, an old Sufi tale,[1] is usually told while the patient is in trance.

> "One day, a long time ago, in Persia, the Mulla Nasrudin was walking through the town with a group of followers when a woman [or a man, if the patient is a man] approached them with her hands cupped. She said, 'If you're so clever, tell me if the bird in my hand is alive or dead.' What this woman planned to do was to make herself look smart by making Nasrudin look dumb. If he said 'Alive,' she would squash the bird and show it to be dead. If he said 'Dead,' she would let the bird fly away alive. Nasrudin paused for a moment, looked her in the eye, and said, *'It's in your hands now,'* and walked away."

For a dramatic impact, the therapist can just leave the room and let the patient alert from trance himself or herself.

THE THERAPIST'S PERSONAL POWER

Power has a bad reputation in our culture. For many it conjures up images of dictators and bullies. Yet we all wish power for those who have values with which we agree. When you think of Gandhi or Churchill or Mother Theresa doesn't the phrase "More power to them" strike a receptive chord? When we think of many other leaders we feel glad that they do not have more political power than they do because we do not agree with their vision of the good life. Like political power, personal power can be good or bad depending upon how it is used. Hypnotherapists who bring a sense of personal empowerment into the session and use it to work for the patient's good have a more significant effect than therapists

---

[1]We were told this Sufi tale, so we cannot provide a written source for it.

who do not have such a sense. But if a therapist were to use this ability to communicate personal power only for his or her own ego gratification, or to take advantage of a patient, obviously the patient would be better off if the therapist experienced himself or herself as inept.

Basically, wimps cannot be very good existential therapists. At a critical intuitive level patients will know if the therapist is credible when he or she talks about the courage to be responsible for one's life. A plumber should not be working on someone else's house if his or her own sink is clogged. For existential clinicians, the therapist–patient dialogue is viewed as the most important variable of the therapeutic process. This does not mean that the therapist must share a lot about his or her personal life with the patient. The therapist is there to hear the patient's story, not to share his own or her own. How much self-revelation a therapist engages in depends on the therapist's decisions. The degree of self-revelation should vary from therapist to therapist, and in each therapist–patient relationship. There is no "right" degree of self-revelation. But it is important when the therapist talks about freedom, responsibility, courage, and change that he or she speaks from personal experience.

Three common pitfalls lie in wait for therapists. First, there is the widespread idea that people, especially patients, are very fragile and like fine china can easily shatter. Nothing can be farther from the truth. The overwhelming majority of people (and patients) have very strong defenses. Our techniques are not so powerful that one mistake on our part will send them to the hospital. Second, too many people in our fields (psychology, psychiatry, social work, nursing, and the other healing professions) have a high need to be liked. Sometimes when a professional acts with clarity, determination, and personal empowerment he or she may not seem on the surface to be such "a nice guy." But we believe that patients do better from the beginning if they sense that the therapist working with them is a powerful change agent rather than just a nice person to be around. This is somewhat difficult to describe; the acts of power by a hypnotherapist are subtle, yet critical. The therapist's "need" to be liked by each patient works against the freedom of empowerment.

Third, therapists, in our opinion, rank low when it comes to one issue that we, as existentialists, value highly: therapeutic risk taking. We know therapists who are skydivers, bungee jumpers, race car drivers, or high rollers in the casino; but when it comes to doing psychotherapy, these people are often mundane and predictable. We have observed that the communication of most therapists is often too rigid or too narrow to accommodate the broad array of realities presented to them by patients. Therapists tend to say the same things, do the same things, and present the same old realities to too many patients too often. Such repetition certainly does not help to lower the burn-out rate among therapists.

We were attracted to hypnosis and hypnotherapy in part because of the flexibility afforded to the therapist by working with trance processes. As we often say to patients, "Your imagination and your potentials are only limited by those limits you choose to impose." As Yapko (1990, p. 266) observes, "If the imagination doesn't create new directions, the will doesn't have anyplace to go but around and around." This truth applies to therapists as well as patients. When we train hypnotherapists, we state that the therapist is not engaging in enough risk taking, and therefore is not being powerful enough, if at least once a week he or she is not leaving the therapy room feeling somewhat anxious about having taken the risk to do something new and different with a patient, the outcome of which will not be known for a while. Malpractice suits are a legitimate concern; however, that is why professionals carry malpractice insurance. Most of the best psychotherapists we know have had to deal with this issue as part of the price of being good. Too many patients are "addicted" to safety. A therapist who is limited in the same way as the patient cannot be helpful.

HYPNOSIS AND SELF-HYPNOSIS AS TOOLS FOR PERSONAL POWER

We employ a number of hypnotic techniques, especially those using visual imagery, to help patients develop their sense of personal empowerment. However, even without the other techniques, hypnosis and self-hypnosis are effective tools toward that therapeutic end. Hypnosis is an exercise in focused attention. All acts of power require focused attention. In the martial arts it is focused attention that centers "the will" that allows a small woman to break cement bricks with the side of her hand or her elbow. As Rollo May (1969, p. 220) stated, "When we analyze will . . . we shall find ourselves pushed back to the level of attention or intention as the seat of will. The effort which goes into the exercise of the will is really effort of attention; the strain in willing is the effort to keep consciousness clear, i.e., the strain of keeping the attention focused."

When we give patients the directive to practice self-hypnosis each day, it is a directive to practice the art of focusing and refocusing with their attention. As May stated, this effort of attention is really an exercise of the will or of will-power. One of our clearest observations after years of working intimately with thousands of people is that this skill, the skill of learning to focus, generalizes to other realms. Once patients learn and practice staying focused in their hypnotic work, they can usually learn to do so in the areas of life they came to work on in therapy. Again, hypnosis becomes therapeutic in and of itself, in addition to any other specific clinical techniques used with the trance.

Another advantage of regularly using the directive to do self-hypnosis is that it requires effort for the patient to take the time to do it every day. Some people love doing self-hypnosis and say it is the best part of each day, but after a while most patients find the routine somewhat boring. As every psychotherapist knows, growth requires an effort. Habit is easy; change is difficult. There is a sign in our office that says, "Practice what is best and habit will render it easiest." In *The Road Less Traveled* (one of the few trade books we recommend to patients) M. Scott Peck (1978, p. 85) says, "The act of extending one's limits implies effort. One extends one's limits only by exceeding them, and exceeding limits requires effort." Therefore, practicing something such as self-hypnosis that requires effort because it is not always interesting and because its positive results are not directly apparent is practice of a healthy process. Such effort or discipline is usually required for the patient to make therapeutic changes. Just as in the case of focusing attention, this skill generalizes from the specific task of making an effort by doing the self-hypnosis every day to a general way of being-in-the-world. The patient becomes a more powerful person when he or she is willing to make the necessary effort to achieve objectives.

There are other reasons that hypnosis and self-hypnosis in and of themselves can help promote personal empowerment. As we stated earlier, the language of hypnosis can be reduced to the simple terms of a when–then message. *When* patients alter their existential reality by "buying" the when–then message presented by the therapist, *then* they can achieve a successful outcome. For example, "*When* you do your self-hypnosis, *then* you will become alert; you will feel slightly more determined and slightly more able to stand up to your children and enforce reasonable limits." These messages are not limited to self-hypnosis. However, self-hypnosis is a good example to use because it is something that every patient can do if he or she is willing to make the effort. This directive can also be very helpful as a diagnostic indicator in that self-hypnosis, while it often gets routine, is relatively easy to do. It requires 15 minutes a day, and can be carried out in any place at any time of day. If the patient will not follow this most simple and nonthreatening of all the directives we give, a successful outcome for his or her therapy is doubtful.

A few years ago the C.E.O. of one of this country's largest corporations come to us for help. He wanted to stop smoking. We had a successful outcome in just one session. The success prompted the patient, whom we will call Bob, to fly to Pittsburgh from New York in his private jet every other week for a 2-hour session to work on some of his interpersonal issues. But after the third 2-hour session we terminated therapy because this patient refused to follow the directive to do self-hypnosis daily. During this third session he said, "Look, I know you can't understand this but my day and your day are just not the same." He was attempting to communicate how busy he was. At the end of this session as he was walking out of the office the therapist said, "Just one last point,

Bob. You're wrong about something you said today. Both of our days are exactly the same. We start at midnight with 24 hours and we each decide what to do with that time." Two weeks later he called to make another appointment, at which point he admitted that he was now doing his directed self-hypnosis work each day. Without that effort on his part it is unlikely the therapeutic work could have succeeded.

VISUAL IMAGERY

It seems likely that any practitioner of hypnotherapy from the existential perspective will use a lot of visual imagery in his or her practice. Visual imagery allows patients to experience new behaviors in a way that is more safe and comfortable than actually doing these new behaviors in the outside world. Everyone who has studied psychology knows that the use of imagery and mental rehearsal is valuable for many patients. But no one really knows why or how it works. The explanations probably lie within the relatively new field of brain research, where, as the well-known researcher Marvin Minsky from M.I.T. told one of us in a private conversation just a few years ago, "We are just coming out of the dark ages and most of our ideas are probably wrong."

Even though we have no definite idea why the use of visual imagery works in clinical hypnotherapy, patients seem to respond better if they think we and they themselves understand the why and the how. Since our job is to alter the existential reality of the patient in ways that are helpful, we act like the wise father who pointed to any rabbit in the cage when answering the child's question, "Which is mine?" This is not to say that our explanation to our patients about how visual imagery works is not true. We are just not experts in brain research and are not as up to date as we should be in this rapidly changing field. Our current understanding comes from the work of Bennett (1989) and Rumelhard (1989). They say that a memory is a pattern of electrical impulses across the brain (from neuron receptor to neuron receptor). Since there are millions of receptors on the brain surface, there are an infinite number of possible patterns, each representing a thought or memory. When we produce an imaginary image of an event as if it were really happening, we create the same electrical pattern in the brain that would occur if the event were actually happening. At that moment the brain does not know the difference.[2] When we engage in repeated mental rehearsals of an event we create habitual neurological links, which in the manner of habits begin almost automatically to repeat themselves.[3]

We do not know how valid this theory is or even how much of it is supported or undermined by current research. What we do know is that this explanation seems to meet the needs of our patients. It is sophisticated enough to sound logical and simple enough to be understood. Some patients do not need this kind of explanation: they just do the work. Other patients habitually block their own growth with the defense of overintellectualization. For those patients we will often process and work through this defense rather than give an explanation of our work. But there are some patients who ask in a healthy, curious way how the hypnotic work we are using with them works, and it seems rude not to offer them an explanation. The phrase "We aren't sure" would not meet their needs. With these patients we use the explanation just outlined.

All people who do visual imagery do so in trance. If you watch for physical evidence of trance, such as the stillness of their body or the change in their breathing, or if you question them about their experience of the passage of time, there can be no doubt about their trance state. Visual imagery can (and often is) accomplished just by asking the patient or subject to produce a certain image. The professional literature is full of discussion about the use of imagery, and most of this literature does not mention hypnosis or trance. It is our expe-

---

[2]This is why the subject needs to be directed to engage the event from their viewpoint as if it were happening as opposed to seeing themselves doing it as if on television.

[3]According to Bennett (1989), the same may be true for talking to yourself about an event or writing about an event.

rience that formal trance induction before the clinical imagery begins makes the experience "more real" for most patients, and therefore seems to produce better clinical results. We strongly recommend a formal hypnotic induction before starting clinical work using visual imagery. Moreover, a percentage of the population (we estimate about 30%) have trouble producing visual imagery. Using a trance induction usually facilitates the ability to create visual images; that is, while in trance these subjects can usually get an image they initially were unable to experience.

The best way to enhance patients' sense of personal empowerment is to get them to do something, anything, that they previously believed they could not do. Milton Erickson always talked about getting patients to take a step, *however small*, in *any* direction, as the beginning of therapeutic change. This process can be greatly encouraged by having the patient visualize a desired outcome or new behavior. This is first done in the safety of trance in our office, with our guidance and encouragement. Later, this "mental rehearsal" becomes part of the patient's "homework" or self-hypnosis directive. This use of visual imagery to encourage new behaviors is part of our existential hypnotherapy for almost all of our patients.

Visual imagery also has a diagnostic purpose. If a patient cannot even imagine himself or herself engaging in a new behavior, then you have probably asked him or her to take too big a step at one time. But sometimes there is a strong secondary gain in maintaining the patient's lack of progress, a topic we will address in Chapter 6.

POWER ANCHORS

If having a patient imagine a desired outcome increases the probability that he or she will be able to achieve that outcome (and it usually does), than the metaphoric icing on the cake is to associate a feeling of being powerful with that visual image. The best way to do that is to use "anchoring," a technique developed by Bandler and Grinder (1979). Of all the work detailed by this pair, this technique is by far the most important to hypnotherapists with an existential orientation. Any practitioner not familiar with the work of Bandler and Grinder who is familiar with basic research in learning and knows the term "paired associate" should be very comfortable with the logistics of this technique.

Early in our hypnotic work with a patient, while he or she is in trance, and while we are giving some of the standard messages that we give to almost every patient, we say something like the following:

> "Frank, you have many experiences as part of your personal history that will help you do the work you came here to do; some we have already talked about. Of all these experiences probably the most important group or set of experiences are all the times in your life when you attempted to do something and it came out just the way you wanted it to, maybe even surprisingly better than you had hoped. Times when you felt powerful, competent, on top of the world, like there was nothing you couldn't do. Now sometimes you had one of these moments but it only lasted for a short while before someone came along and said or did something to ruin the feeling; but that was okay, since you still had those few moments. Maybe the good feelings lasted all day. Sometimes when people remember one of these moments they remember a childhood experience and say to themselves that it was unimportant, but those moments and feelings are important too. Now I would like you to remember one of these moments. It doesn't need to be the best one ever, just one time when you felt for a moment like there was nothing you couldn't do. When you remember one of these moments please let me know by nodding your head."

When the patient lets you know through a phenomenological or self-description (in this case, by nodding the head) that he or she is visualizing such a positive moment, and when you can see bodily changes in the patient that confirm an experience of empowerment (these changes include sitting up slightly with shoulders back and breathing deeper and higher up in chest), you then ask the patient to deepen this experience by using all his or her senses: to see the things he or she *saw* at that time, even if those images are vague; to pay attention to what he or she *heard*, including the things he or she said to himself or herself; and most of all to remember what he or she *felt* at that time. As all this happens and as you, the clinician, become aware that the patient is now reliving (and most especially feeling) a moment of his or her personal empowerment, you should create an association for this moment by means of some stimulus that you can later reproduce. We usually use a firm touch or grasp of the patient's shoulder (we always get permission to touch before we begin our hypnotic work). If you do not want to touch the patient, an auditory stimulus such as snapping your fingers or clapping your hands works just as well. After about a minute we will ask the patient to erase this memory of empowerment from his or her mind and we move on with other trance work. We will repeat this pairing of one stimulus and the patient's feeling of power a couple of times a session for the first few weeks of our work, usually asking the patient to remember a different experience each time if he or she can.

After a few weeks of this procedure a link or association is established between the patient's feeling of empowerment and the stimuli that the therapist can reproduce. Next, we will have the patient engage in mental rehearsals using trance and visual imagery in the office. While the patient is imagining himself or herself engaging in a new desired behavior, we will "fire" the appropriate stimulus. Now the patient is not only imagining himself or herself engaging in this new behavior (which in and of itself is helpful) but he or she is feeling powerful while doing so. This system significantly increases the probability that the patient will be able to engage in this positive behavior out of the office in his or her life-world.

The hypnotherapist must help the patient to get in touch with moments of empowerment in his or her history by communicating the request to do so in a congruent manner. The therapist needs to raise his or her voice and the tempo of the spoken words to match the request. It is not helpful to ask the patient to remember this type of experience while using the same calm, low, relaxed voice that most of us use during a hypnotic induction. If the patient cannot remember even one moment in his or her entire life when he or she felt empowered, probably he or she needs to be treated for clinical depression. Almost all patients can remember such positive moments. But some need time to think about their empowering moments; we often direct these people to go back over picture albums to help recall positive life experiences.

This technique is so effective in helping patients remember their own history of empowerment and then using those positive feelings to promote therapeutic growth that we set up this association of the feeling of personal power and a stimulus that we can reproduce and utilize it for almost every patient as part of our existential hypnotherapy. This technique is also very effective for these relatively rare moments when we work with patients outside the office. For example, one of us was hired to work with a college football team. The kicker, a much-sought-after high school star, was unable to feel confident in critical game situations and had cost the team victories by missing field goals late in close games. The hypnotherapy work with this player consisted of visual imagery and the establishment of a power anchor produced by touching his elbow in a certain manner. During the game, just before this kicker was about to go onto the field to attempt a field goal, the therapist (who was working for the team and was on the sidelines with the players) would talk to the player, reminding him to take a deep breath. Simultaneously, out of the player's conscious awareness, the therapist would grab his elbow, firing this established power anchor to increase his confidence level at this critical moment. (Players were always being grabbed by the coaches while they were being talked to, so this seemed a matter-of-fact behavior.[4])

[4]Students of psychotherapy are usually upset that textbooks almost always are limited to cases that have successful outcomes. We proudly report this case to be a dramatic failure. The kicker was eventually demoted to second and third string and spent his last 2 years "on the

There are patients who cannot identify any powerful memories in their history and need the hypnotherapist's help to experience a powerful feeling. Some depressed patients have absolutely no idea what it means to feel powerful or masterful. At these times the therapist and the patient must work together creatively to generate a powerful feeling that can be used as a power anchor. Sometimes it is helpful to simply ask a patient during trance to *imagine* herself as powerful within a particular context relevant to that person. Once the patient generates an image of power, she can be asked to pay close attention to exactly how she looks, including the posture of her body and the look on her face, to how she is breathing, and to how she is talking and behaving. Often, it is helpful to give the patient a directive to examine this image for a few minutes every day during self-hypnosis; in essence, the examination becomes a process of mentally rehearsing that pattern of experience or behavior. Some patients may require an explanation as to just what it means to behave powerfully; thus the therapist might need to model this pattern for the patient or let the patient choose a powerful model, real or fictional, and then simulate the model. Bandler and Grinder (1979) refer to this latter strategy as use of a "referential index shift."

Sometimes we ask a patient who is confused about what it is like to be and feel powerful to stand up, clasp hands with the therapist, and push as the therapist does the same. The patient can then be prompted to yell "No!" while the therapist yells "Yes!," or to yell "Yes!" as the therapist yells "No!" Other words or phrases can be substituted—for example, the patient can say the existential words "I will!" while the therapist says "You won't!" Once the patient seems to be experiencing his or her power, the therapist can create an associated anchor for that feeling.

---

bench." One of the major lessons learned by the authors was that this was an inappropriate case to accept since it was clear from the onset that this player resented seeing a "shrink" and was doing so only to follow the coach's order. He rarely did his self-hypnosis and mental rehearsal as directed.

One can help a passive, powerless patient by making use of the concept from gestalt theory that all experience exists on a continuum with polar opposites such as sad–happy, passive–aggressive, dependent–independent, or humility–arrogance. Many patients with clinical problems can best be understood as being stuck close to or at a particular polar extreme. For example, many depressed patients are overly passive and also overly dependent. Gestalt therapists believe that the healthy or fully functioning person is in touch with and has access to both polarities of the various continuums of human experience and that such persons can flexibly slide along these continuums to be wherever in experience a particular life context demands. This framework can be utilized to help a patient who has been lacking in life experiences of a powerful nature. Even if a person is stuck at one end of a continuum of experience, such as passivity, he or she is at least *on* that continuum and therefore has the *potential* to experience the polar opposite of that experience, as well as the potential to experience all the in-between states that exist on that continuum. Whether or not such gestalt concepts are valid is not as important as our finding that most patients will "buy into" these concepts when they are explained in a simple, logical manner. In so doing, these patients have begun to admit or be invested in the reality that other powerful potentials exist for them.

Once a patient seems to understand the gestalt idea of continuums, it can be utilized hypnotherapeutically to increase personal empowerment. We had a patient named Steve who was very shy and passive and seemingly unable to assert himself even in small ways. The following excerpt from a hypnotic session with Steve reveals the use of gestalt concepts to empower him:

"Steve, before you let go into hypnotic trance, we discussed and you seemed to understand, that you have been stuck at the shy and the passive ends of the shy–bold and the passive–aggressive continuums. That means that the potential to choose to be bold and aggressive exists within you. What I'd like you to do now, Steve, is get a picture or image on one side of your mind of yourself looking shy and passive, and nod your head when you see that image."

When the patient indicates that he has found or created the desired image, ask him on what side of his mind he sees it. Then ask him to tell you exactly what he sees. Next ask the patient to become or to role-play that image, looking like the image as much as possible, and even feeling how the person in the image feels. The first image we call for portrays the "unwanted" or problematic experience or behavior, since most patients can more easily conjure up this image and then experience it because it has been their more common or habitual way of being-in-the-world. When the patient seems to access the feeling associated with the image, set up an anchor to that feeling state. In Steve's case, a light touch on his right shoulder (he saw the image of himself as shy and passive on the right side of his mind) was used to anchor his shy, passive feelings. We used a light touch because it was congruent with the type of feelings that were being dealt with here. At this point, the therapist said: "Steve, now on the left side of your mind, please get an image of yourself as bold and aggressive and nod your head when you see that picture."

We have discovered that following these steps, of first explaining gestalt polarities and continuum model, and then directing the patient to create an image of the habitual, problematic experience, facilitates the patient's ability to access a desired or more powerful image. However, some patients may still need help getting this image; strategies we discussed earlier, such as using a referential index, can be utilized to help them. After Steve nodded his head, he was asked to become and to talk like that more powerful image, and the therapist firmly grasped his left shoulder. At this point, it can be very helpful to allow the patient to role-play a dialogue between these two "parts" or potentials of himself. Such a dialogue can address the patient's view regarding being-in-the-world in these different ways. The therapist helped Steve to experience these potentials by applying the relevant anchor for the different feeling states during the dialogue. Even though the procedures just described might seem to reinforce the more habitual and problematic feelings or behaviors, the structure, focus, and compartmentalization that is involved in this process seems to help many patients get in touch with desired experiences that will increase their personal power. To defuse resistance to change and to communicate the value we place on it, we also usually explain to patients that *all* parts or potentials of the person can be helpful or healthy, depending on the situation or context that the person finds himself or herself in.

After the above hypnotic session, a power anchor for the bold, aggressive feelings Steve imaged was used to help Steve become more assertive in his world.

SELF-POWER ANCHORS

Besides those power anchors that are applied by hypnotherapists to evoke powerful feelings in patients, there are also anchors that patients can utilize by themselves.

One category of these self-power anchors are behaviors or rituals that a patient can easily reproduce, such as taking a deep breath of air, squeezing the thumb to the middle finger, or both. The strategy of taking a deep breath and squeezing two fingers is a focused attention strategy that can help panic disorder patients feel more in control at the onset of an attack. When this strategy is paired or associated with a powerful memory, it becomes a self-power anchor that can be reproduced by the patient. We often will ask the patient during trance to take a deep breath at the same time that he or she is remembering powerful moments and while we are setting up a power anchor. Then we suggest to the patient that he or she can access power anytime at all just by taking a deep breath. Cues or stimuli such as the word "Power!" that the patient can say in his or her own mind or out loud can be utilized in similar ways.

Another category of self-power anchors are *imaged power objects*, images that have been associated with power for the patient. A particular image can already be a part of the patient's history, but it can be made more empowering if the therapist links it to a feeling of power during trance. For example, one patient who loved railroad trains spontaneously used the metaphorical image of a diesel locomotive while making a point about power to the hypnotherapist. Later, the therapist suggested to the patient that he see this image in one corner of his mind while the patient was remembering a powerful moment. After that, the patient was able to access power by imaging the locomotive in the same corner of his mind or visual field.

A similar technique, derived from anthropological and mythological sources (see Feinstein & Krippner, 1988; Harner, 1990), is the use of *power animals*. Here the image of a particular animal that the patient associates with power can be utilized to help that patient access power when it is needed.

Finally, *tangible power objects,* such as totems and charms, can be put to good use. These have been described extensively in the anthropological literature and in one of our earlier works, *The Courage to Recover* (King et al., 1989). We often give patients a directive to select and bring to therapy a small object in their possession or one they can obtain that they ordinarily do not carry around that they already associate with power in some way or that makes sense to them as a power object. A piece of jewelry, a stone, or even a pine cone might be examples of such objects. Then during trance, and while the patient has the object on his or her person, the therapist can establish an association between the object and the feeling of power. Often we will ask the person to continue to bring the power object to therapy, to have it on his or her person during self-hypnosis, and, of course, to have it whenever that person chooses to be powerful in the world.

DIRECTIVES—GO FLY A PLANE

A 35-year-old male patient once came in suffering from mild depression and complaining that he felt "stuck and unhappy in his life." He was a professional who felt unappreciated and underpaid by his boss and his family. He also wanted help in losing weight. During intake, he said that he always wanted to fly an airplane but had not yet gotten around to taking flying lessons. After 3 weeks therapy was suspended for a month while the therapist took summer vacation. The patient was directed to contact a flight instructor and to spend at least 2 hours a week during the month on flying lessons. When the therapist returned after his vacation, the patient had spent so many hours on his ground and air instruction that he was already ready to solo for the first time. In fact, 2 weeks later, when he did a solo flight, he experienced it as the most powerful moment in his life and later relived it during an anchoring exercise. In about 4 months' time this patient was discharged from psychotherapy after having made significant, positive changes in many aspects of his life including all the areas he initially complained about.

In the workshops we teach on hypnotherapy, cases like this one often draw questions and criticism from participants. We are often asked what business we had to direct this patient's leisure activities, especially in this case, where the directive was expensive and even slightly dangerous. In answer, we reply that it is important to note that the patient volunteered the information that *he* always wanted to take lessons. His failure to do so was another indication of "stuckness" or lack of movement toward a desired goal. More importantly, as existentialists, we understand a person's life-world to operate as a gestalt or totally interdependent unit. The work life, the family life, the sex life, the health issues in life, the recreational part of life, and so on—each influences all the others. A sense of personal achievement or empowerment in one area of life to some degree always carries over to other aspects of life. Good hypnotherapy can increase this carry over effect of empowerment even more.

As Rollo May (1969) details, "Will power is desire plus action." Everyone wants a good life. Some people are willing to work for it, but others just wish for it. Too often the psychotherapy process gets stuck in words. In fact, often psychotherapy actually enables the patient not to take a risk or make the hard effort because, after all, he or she believes that he or she is working on the problem by talking about it in therapy; therefore, family and friends should be patient with his

or her neurotic behaviors. Existential hypnotherapy encourages and requires the patient to move forward in his or her
life-world now. "Nothing succeeds like success" may be a
simple and even trite saying, but it is nevertheless true.

Directives are very important for hypnotherapy because
we usually see patients just once a week (sometimes every
other week). When the patient follows a therapist's directive
between sessions, this is a way of maintaining the existential
presence of the therapist for the patient between sessions and
dramatically intensifies the therapeutic work. Moreover, if
directives take up enough of the patient's time or are unpleasant enough, they can motivate a degree of clinical success just
so the patient can end therapy (Haley, 1984).

The most common directive we use—in fact, we use it
with almost every patient—is the directive for what we call
"self-hypnosis." Earlier we discussed how from our theoretical perspective, almost all hypnosis is dual hypnosis and is really part of the therapist–patient dialogue. However, to simplify things we label this process self-hypnosis when we talk
about it with the patient. This directive has five major therapeutic uses. First, it deepens and enhances the cooperative
relationship between the hypnotherapist and the patient. It
is an easy directive to follow (it takes just 12 to 15 minutes a
day) and each time the patient does it, he or she is "proving"
to himself or herself how cooperative and willing to work he
or she is, a great self-fulfilling prophecy. Second, the practice
of trance deepens the ability to use it. Like any other skill, it
improves with practice. Third, self-hypnosis itself becomes a
part of a when–then hypnotic message: "*When* you do the self-
hypnosis, *then* you'll feel the urge to overeat [or whatever]
reduced."

A fourth advantage of having the patient practice self-
hypnosis is that later you can easily add mental rehearsals or
other visualization work to this directive. For example, "This
week when you do your self-hypnosis, after you get to your
favorite place I want you to . . . [whatever]." The fifth and
last major value of this directive is that it has an important
diagnostic function, vis-à-vis the prognosis for successful
hypnotherapy. It is easy for a therapist to make a mistake in

judgment about what a patient is capable of doing when giving behavioral directives, especially early in the therapy process. A self-hypnosis directive is one that almost all patients can do if they are willing to take the time and make any effort at all. If a patient does not follow this directive regularly he or she is either not willing to work hard enough for the therapy to have any chance of success or is very ambivalent about getting better. The therapist would need to assess which of these is the operative explanation: in the first case, to terminate therapy, and in the later case, to deal with the patient's ambivalence.

Aside from the self-hypnosis directive, we usually use other behavioral directives in our hypnotherapy work. It is often very difficult to get the patient moving when complex psychodynamics are involved, such as important secondary gains that may be associated with symptoms. This is why we often begin with behavioral directives that are relevant to the patient, but not directly related to the reason he or she entered hypnotherapy. Directing the patient to learn to fly an airplane is a case in point. Another common example is directing a patient to lose weight, to stop smoking, or begin to exercise. (Again, this is the case when these are not the presenting problems.) We tell the patients that they are lucky that they have a bad habit. At this time, they usually look at us as if they think we are crazy, but we do have their full attention. We then continue by telling them that it often takes a long time in psychotherapy to raise one's self-esteem and help a person feel more empowered. Yet correcting a bad habit can accomplish these goals almost overnight. Since they often will have wanted to begin to exercise regularly and lose 15 pounds anyway, this directive to do so will not only help them with that issue, but will also speed up the hypnotherapy process.

We encourage patients to stand up to bosses or family members, take a trip alone if they have never done so, read 1 hour a night rather than watching television, enroll in and complete an art class, and so on. All these small changes are not the desired outcome of our clinical work, but rather an important part of the process. We help patients engage in these new behaviors by using visualization and mental rehearsal paired with power anchor, as well as congruently communicating to them that we know they can do it, and that we expect them to do it. Most important, we give them the when–then hypnotic message that when they do this they will then be more aware than ever before of their ability to take charge of their lives, the living definition of a sense of empowerment.

Anxiety Management

As we stated in Chapter 1, existentialism views anxiety as a fundamental condition of human existence. Embracing this condition—as opposed to denying or fighting it—is a necessary aspect of healthy living. As people go through the world they are commonly presented with the choice of staying on the same path or of taking the risk to explore new paths. Sameness, even if boring or uncomfortable, at least feels safe when contrasted with the unknown. One of our earlier books, *The Courage to Recover* (King et al., 1989), concludes that many clients in counseling who are suffering from the pain, depression, boredom, or rage associated with current life contexts *already know* the changes they should make, but feel too anxious and thus are paralyzed about making or even tentatively exploring change. That earlier book concluded that often all people need is the *courage* to make needed changes. Often it is helpful to teach clients that they are *choosing* to participate in particular life contexts that are uncomfortable—whether it be a job, or a marriage, or whatever—and that the anxiety they experience when thinking about possible change is a necessary aspect of the growth process and should not be seen as a signal to withdraw into feelings of being stuck or powerless.

To most people, the word "anxiety" connotes something tense, uncomfortable, or scary. Anxiety is something to be avoided or circumvented no matter what effort is needed. Many people stay in a relationship or on a job, or do not speak their piece with a spouse, boss, or colleague, just because they do not want to "rock the boat." They will do whatever it takes to avoid dreaded anxiety. Sometimes such people stay in therapy because their anxiety grows whenever termination is discussed. They would prefer to stay with the Valium, the Xanax, the Prozac, the lithium, or the whatever. But at what cost? Most of us know people close to us who have literally "sold their soul" to avoid some discomfort.

We recognize that severe or intense anxiety can be incapacitating. In some cases measures such as anxiolytics are indicated to enable the patient to function well enough to explore his or her realities and the choices available. Some patients need help in reducing their extreme anxiety before they even become secure and attentive enough to sit and listen to the idea that they have choices they can make and the freedom to make them. Existentialists recognize that choice is always available to human beings. Although the choices we may have before us may not be the choices we desire, *there are always choices*. Existentialists, instead of viewing anxiety as a destructive and threatening experience, see it as a signal portending the potential to increase personal power and awareness of the self by taking responsibility for making choices about one's path. Some patients are overwhelmed with anxiety because right from the start of their lives they were rarely given any choices to make, were never recognized by others as having any power to make a choice (and therefore never learned to recognize such power within themselves), and therefore feel totally powerless and at the mercy of the external world and its forces. Given that kind of background, of course, they are anxious. Wouldn't you be? Examples of such people would include those who were physically or sexually abused while young, or those overprotected or enmeshed in symbiotic relationships through their formative years. Such people—those who were never given any choices or supported in being powerful—often do not know that they have the freedom to make choices. Sometimes they need help, in the form of medication or a safer environment, such as a hospital, just to sit still long enough and be focused enough to hear someone tell them that they do have the power to make choices.

Often the therapist can help anxious clients just by explaining some of the existential realities about anxiety we have mentioned in this text. Relabeling anxiety, giving it a more positive and less debilitating meaning, can change a client's perspective and help that client to accept the risks of exploring change. We have discovered that the existential perspective on anxiety is an exciting and productive viewpoint for patients as well as clinicians. Too often, however, a clinician has an intellectual understand of this concept, yet does not really grasp it. The clinician needs to really embrace this reality and experience it himself or herself in order to adequately communicate this framework to patients and effectively utilize it clinically. In other words, clinicians need to *relabel* their own anxiety in a productive way and let it fuel their own explorations of personal potentials and power. For example, when you were last consulted by a patient with a unique or strange pattern of symptoms, did you get anxious or "bummed out," and did you curse the referral source? Or did you feel *excited* about the opportunity to learn and be creative and discover more about yourself by treating this difficult case? All psychotherapy is, to some degree, an education process, and all therapists are teachers. The potentially positive relationship between anxiety and healthy living is one of the more important "lessons" patients need to learn. Since hypnotic trance involves a subtle suspension of ordinary conscious frameworks and an increased openness to new realities, we usually communicate early during trance the potential for new comfortable experiences and realities. We often remind our patients of Kierkegaard's (1944, pp. 138–139) wise words, including "He who is schooled in anxiety is schooled in potentiality" and "Anxiety is always to be understood as oriented toward freedom."

EXISTENTIAL ANXIETY AS AN EXPLANATION FOR CLINICAL PROBLEMS

In Chapter 1, we pointed out that all existential thinkers and clinicians view the reality of freedom, choice, and responsibility as central to healthy human experience. We also pointed out that clinical work involves helping clients to realize that they are volunteers in, and not just victims of, their life circumstances. *They are responsible* and have choices. Usually anxiety arises when people begin to "own" their freedom. As children get older they are faced with the prospect of making their own choices and taking responsibility for themselves. We are all aware of the anxiety associated with adolescence and young adulthood, when people are faced with this increased responsibility. High rates of alcoholism, drug abuse, depression, and suicide are associated with the significant level of anxiety experienced during this phase of the life cycle. The developmental theme of the adolescent passage is an identity crisis (Erikson, 1968) associated with the anxiety of deciding "Who am I?" and "How will I fit in?," which, of course interfaces with the existential anxiety of new freedom, choice, and responsiblity. Counseling young people often involves teaching them to have a more comfortable understanding of the anxiety associated with this new freedom so that the effort does not become paralyzing. In fact, the therapist should teach the adolescent to use anxiety as energy to motivate him or her to take healthy risks and explore potentials and choices. Concomitant to the process of such healthy exploration and decision making is self-empowerment.

Many clinicians have discovered that growing up—which existentialists might define as assuming increasing responsiblity for ourselves and the situations we find ourselves in—is a neverending process. Most adolescents and young adults normally go through the critical, anxiety-producing passage into adulthood with relatively minor difficulties. For some, however, this passage is delayed or totally blocked. Some people will live a life of relative sameness, continuing to live with their parents until later years or substituting surrogate parents, perhaps in the form of a structured and safe military career or marriage with a parentlike caretaking mate. Such people sacrifice freedom and the ability to manifest their potentials for the safety of sameness, structure, and protection from making choices. Two potential problems are associated with inability to face anxiety of freedom associated with becoming independent. First, the safe structure often collapses: parents die or become disabled, the caretaking mate decides he or she is tired of being a surrogate parent and leaves, and jobs disappear. The second problem is that sameness over time often bores and depresses the human spirit. Even though anxiety is associated with freedom, choice, and responsibility, it is also associated with an increased sense of power and excitement when we do make active choices about our lives and take responsibility for ourselves. Patients must face the fact that an inability to make such active choices tends to lead to feelings of powerlessness and depression. Therapists' caseloads are full of people who feel depressed because they are "stuck" in situations where they may be very safe and secure, but feel deprived of power and excitement. When therapists point out the choices available to such clients, they will commonly complain of their "anxiety" or fear about even exploring alternative life choices.

Existentially oriented therapists will always frame life as offering exciting choices or opportunities to explore and to discover one's potentials. An existentially oriented person will tend to feel dissatisfied with sameness or with conventional patterns (Fagen & Shepherd, 1970).

In Chapter 3 we described the use of a variety of gestalt therapy techniques within a hypnotic framework. We discussed the close similarity of hypnotic and gestalt strategies because the latter are themselves naturalistic trance experiences. We also discussed how formal trance induction can increase therapeutic results with these techniques. Gestalt therapists are existentially oriented (Van Dusen, 1960), and view anxiety not as an unwanted experience to be gotten rid of but as an indication of potentials or aspects of the person to be explored.

We like Simkin's (1976, p. 17) theoretical perspective on the personality: Simkin argues that personality is not like an onion with layers to be peeled away (with the inner layers accounting for unconscious behavior of which we are unaware), but instead like a rubber ball that has a thick outer layer and is empty inside. Simkin states that this ball floats so that only a portion is exposed while the rest is beneath the surface of the water. What is below the surface is unconscious to the person and yet contains potentials that could be helpful to him or her depending on the context. Anxiety might occur if such potential experiences or patterns of behavior threaten to come to the surface. Therapy can be conceived as experimentation and exploration with these potentials to make them more easily available.

In Chapter 3 we discussed a variety of techniques for "letting go" of excessive anxiety and other problematic feelings. In the remainder of this chapter we will present other hypnotic strategies. All of these techniques are based on the existential perspectives that anxiety is a necessary ingredient of normal and ongoing life and growth, that anxiety is a "calling card" of emerging potentials, and that a degree of anxiety can actually stimulate and enhance one's life. We do recognize that *excessive* anxiety can be debilitating or paralyzing, and as such needs to be diminished or contained.

We will begin with a discussion of self-hypnosis as a tool for managing excessive anxiety and then present some case studies to illustrate other existential hypnotic strategies.

SELF-HYPNOSIS

As we stated in Chapter 4, we give therapeutic directives for work outside the office to virtually all of our patients. With rare exceptions, every patient we do hypnosis with is directed to do self-hypnosis on a daily or other regular basis. We also suggest, in the form of a *contingency suggestion* (see Erickson & Rossi, 1976a), that *when* the patient does self-hypnosis, *then* he or she will have increased comfort. We also make other suggestions about the healthier and more comfortable realities that can be generated by the unconscious as a result of experiencing trance. In cases of excessive anxiety, we often suggest that patients do self-hypnosis a number of times daily. Generally, we suggest to patients that early morning is the best time to do self-hypnosis so that its benefits will be experienced throughout the rest of the day. The next-best time is late afternoon or early evening, when self-hypnosis will help patients "let go" of excessive anxiety or tension generated during the day so that home life or family time will be more comfortable. For patients experiencing insomnia, we suggest doing self-hypnosis after getting into bed; the self-hypnosis will slow the patient down and generate comfort and facilitate drifting from trance into sleep.

We have found that when patients regularly do self-hypnosis, this activity in and of itself will usually result in reduced stress and anxiety and their related symptoms.

In the following transcript we offer an example of the kinds of directions and suggestions we give to patients about doing self-hypnosis. We make these suggestions first while the patient is in trance and then usually repeat them afterward because some patients have posthypnotic amnesia and others have questions about doing the self-hypnosis.

"Mary, beginning this evening or tomorrow morning, soon after you awaken at the latest, and then every morning, I would like you to do self-hypnosis. The way to do that, Mary, is to do just what you did here today. Take a few deep breaths,[1] close your eyes and imagine the chalkboard and . . . [briefly go over the instructions for the structured induction used with the patient]. I'd like you to do self-hypnosis every morning and every afternoon, after you get home from work, and after you say hello to your family and to then experience trance for 15 minutes or longer each time. When you do self-hypnosis, then you will have increased comfort the rest of the day or evening, and when

---

[1]We start almost all of our trance work by asking the patient to take a few deep breaths. In our directives for self-hypnosis, we also begin with the same request. After a few office sessions of hypnosis coupled with weeks of daily self-hypnosis, these few deep breaths become associated with and become an anchor of the trance experience. When patients become anxious, often they will instinctively take a few deep breaths and unwittingly induce a trance that will reduce their anxiety level. Sometimes we will instruct the patients to take the deep breaths when needed; other patients find the mechanism by themselves.

you do self-hypnosis unconscious activity will be generated to create new, healthier, more comfortable realities for you."

There are two major reasons for using self-hypnosis with patients who suffer from anxiety reactions. First, we couple the self-hypnosis directives with a when–then contingency suggestion. *When* you practice your self-hypnosis, *then* you will experience yourself being calmer and more confident. When–then is the basic linguistic structure of a hypnotic suggestion.

The second therapeutic advantage of having each patient practice self-hypnosis on a regular basis over a long period of time (usually well after the psychotherapy with us ends) is that the self-hypnosis is an exercise in focusing on the present. It provides the same healthy learning experience one gets if one practices meditation on a regular basis. Anxiety (and all worry) is anticipatory; it concerns something we fear *in the future*. In the present, in our immediate specific moments, we all feel safe. By having to focus on the present, specific moment—then the next present, specific moment, and so on—most patients eliminate negative anticipatory thoughts and feelings. There is not a magical translation from trance practice to the rest of daily living, but there can be progressive learning about the art of staying focused in the present moment. One can be taught at times of stress to refocus on something in the present.

ANXIETY DISORDERS AND PHOBIAS

Phobias and other irrational fears without associated avoidance behaviors are common clinical problems. Hypnosis is a powerful tool that can be helpful in a variety of ways. Many common traditional fear-reducing techniques employ the use of imagery or visualization (see Kroger & Fezler, 1976; Lazarus, 1984; Wright & Wright, 1987), and trance can significantly enhance these processes.

Simply allowing patients, while in trance, to practice or rehearse an upcoming situation they are phobic or anxious about by imagining the situation in a positive way can reduce anxiety. Wright and Wright (1987) call this method of therapy "protected practice" and state that "it is helpful to the individual to be able to practice a new mode of coping in a projected future-time situation, when all complicating contingencies can be safely examined and coping actions rehearsed" (p. 94). In almost all cases when patients suffer from anxiety in a particular situation we will have them experience that situation through the use of imaging in the safety of our office while we employ a power anchor. We also give them directives to "rehearse" by imagining themselves in anxiety-provoking situations during their own self-hypnosis.

When patients present with multiple fears, we usually work on one phobia at a time, beginning with the one that we believe may be the easiest for the patient to conquer. There is nothing like a history of successful change, even in small, seemingly insignificant areas, to get the therapy process moving.

A very important feature of the treatment is that soon after our hypnosis "rehearsals" begin, we encourage—even require—the patient to face his or her fear in actual life. The good news in life is that when people face their fear, it hardly ever is as bad as they fear; the bad news in life is that when people enact their good fantasies they usually find the reality inferior to the imagined version. Therapy means very little if the learning does not translate into changes outside the therapy sessions. Often psychotherapy can become an excuse not to face one's demons: the patient says, "I'm working on my problem. What else can you expect from me?" It is important that therapists, especially when working with patients who have fears and anxieties, do not let such avoidance continue.

It is helpful when you direct patients to face the person or situation that is the cause of their anxiety, that you include in the directive an expectation of some anxiety. It would be highly unusual if hypnotic therapy was so effective that a patient could quickly go from needing to see a therapist about a situation to an experience of total relaxation in the same situation. Often patients will minimize, discredit, or forget their successful therapy work when they feel the first twinge of anxiety. They need to be directed to focus on the *relative* reduction in anxiety levels rather than on the feeling of anxiety itself. This "misdirection," or change in the focus of perception, is a basic tool of existential hypnotherapy.

The use of imagery, especially when enhanced by hypnotic trance, can often help to resolve problems that are otherwise puzzling and confusing when conventional techniques are employed. For example, Lazarus (1984) explains his "step-up" technique by discussing a young woman who complained of confusing anxiety feelings that overwhelmed her after she received a promotion and a raise. Lazarus suggested that she relax and visualize a "step-up" from her promotion and she then realized that her anxiety stemmed from her fears of being possessed or trapped by her job and its larger salary and greater prestige and losing out on other enjoyments she desired. Lazarus states that because of this awareness, the young woman and he were able to logically discuss her situation and arrive at a solution. Although he does not explain his success in terms of an existential orientation, we presume he helped her to relabel her anxiety and opened her eyes to the exciting choices she now had available to her.

Lazarus also utilizes the "step-up" technique with anxious patients by suggesting that they imagine a feared situation one step further along or imagine what might be called a "worst-case scenario" so that they can discover that they can survive the situation, thus reducing their anxiety. A somewhat similar technique is "flooding" or "implosive" therapy (see Hogan & Kirchner, 1967, 1968; Stampfl & Levis, 1967), in which a patient experiences or imagines a very exaggerated version of his or her fear in order to promote desensitization. For example, a patient with an irrational fear of spiders might imagine being covered with thousands of harmless garden spiders. We rarely use this particular technique, but it is clear that for those who do, the procedure is usually faciliatated by the use of hypnotic trance.

PANIC ATTACKS

Patients who suffer severe panic or anxiety attacks require an additional hypnotic technique in their treatment. They need to be told that of course *when* they practice their self-hypnosis exercises and as they continue to work hard in the psychotherapy session, *then* there will be a significant reduction in the number and severity of such attacks. The therapist must, however, let the patients know that attacks will continue to occur for a while. For those attack moments, as part of clinical hypnosis work, the hypnotherapist must give a posthypnotic suggestion that when the patient does X, the attack will subside.

The X can be any quick, focused attention exercise. We often instruct patients to take a deep breath and hold it, at the same time to squeeze a thumb and middle finger together, to focus on the resulting tension (in the chest, fingers, forearms, and so on) for just 2 seconds, and then to simultaneously let go of both, while saying the phrase "Let go" to themselves. This exercise helps patients to turn their attention from the impending attack to the tension–relaxation sequence in their bodies. If the patient believes in the when–then hypnotic suggestion, it will usually happen. We use mental rehearsals for this technique also. Patients in the office will imagine a panic attack about to happen, do technique X, and notice the comfort they feel during the session. We do not direct patients to imagine an attack coming on during their self-hypnosis sessions. This rehearsal is strictly an office technique.

There are two contraindications for the tension–relaxation technique mentioned above. Do not direct physical tightening of the body for any patient with chest pains or a history of any heart condition or for elderly patients. Second, some patients will experience breathing problems as a signal of an impending attack. These people often have a problem taking a deep breath or holding it. For them, we recommend a focus that does not require an attenuation of the breath. For example, such patients can be instructed to close their eyes and go to "a favorite place" in their mind.

A directive we employ for some patients suffering panic attacks is to ask the patient early in therapy to *try* to have a mild to moderate panic attack three or four times daily. Also, we tell the patient that if he or she has a sense that an attack is beginning, to amplify or augment any bodily sensations or feelings associated with the attack. This paradoxical, and typically Ericksonian, directive seems to give patients an increased feeling of power and control in relationship to the panic attacks. The word "try" is purposeful here since it implies that the patient might "try" to bring on, but not necessarily be successful in bringing on, an attack. Sometimes we will ask a patient to try to have a panic attack while with us in the office. If the patient is successful in starting an attack, we will then suggest that the patient try to amplify whatever bodily sensations he or she is feeling. Quite consistently, when patients amplify these sensations, the feelings will begin to disappear. We believe that panic attacks occur when patients become aware of cues, especially bodily cues, that they have learned to associate with an impending attack, and that they consequently become tense and anxious about the feared attack, which brings on the very attack that is feared. Panic attacks, therefore, seem to have a significant "self-fulfilling" aspect. Again, the directive to purposely try to have attacks or to augment sensations of a beginning attack enables the patient to develop a sense of power and control about these attacks, such that the problem will begin to disappear.

We also believe that it is useful to discover, if possible, if there was an identifiable cause for a patient's first panic attack. Such causes might include not eating breakfast with resulting hypoglycemia (all panic attack patients should be checked for hypoglycemia) or being overcome by fumes in a garage. The first attack for a number of patients is often caused by an absolutely terrifying experience and may have involved loss of consciousness and/or loss of bodily functions; such experiences often generate a one-trial learning in which certain bodily cues that occurred at the time of the attack are associated with fear of an impending attack. After this first learning, similar cues, such as feeling lightheaded when climbing stairs, can trigger fear or anxiety that can increase that feeling and produce a full-scale attack. When the reasons for the patient's first attack can be identified and when the processes just described are explained to the patient, this provides increased control and goes a long way to solving the problem.

Before completing this discussion on panic attacks, we would like to mention our dismay at the proliferation of clinics for treating "panic attack" or "agoraphobia with panic attack" patients and our sorrow that hundreds of thousands of such patients are maintained on anxiolytic drugs such as Xanax or Valium. While we recognize that many people have received help with this paralyzing anxiety or panic through use of such treatments, we wonder how many others have been deprived of their power and their potentials to overcome obstacles by the negative effects of being labeled "agoraphobic" or by the sedating effect of popping a pill in their mouth.

SUBMODALITIES OF EXPERIENCE

Recent developments in neurolinguistic programming (NLP) "submodality" work by Bandler (1985) and some of his associates (Andreas & Andreas, 1987) is of interest in relation to hypnotic work to reduce or manage anxiety. Bandler and Grinder (1979) helped to popularize the concept of representational systems of experience and have pointed out that experience is mostly registered by the *visual, auditory,* and *kinesthetic* systems. (Subhuman species utilize the olfactory and gustatory systems far more than humans.) Furthermore, most people rely on one system in a primary way, which is that person's "primary representational system." Discerning a person's primary system, for example, through that person's word usage (for example, a person who primarily uses words or phrases like "tune into," "sounds like," "I hear you," and so forth, use the auditory system as a primary system), and then utilizing that same system in communication can be very helpful.

Submodalities are elements of experience that can be utilized to change a person's subjective realities and thus generate increased comfort. Submodalities are the elements that can be modulated within any one representational system— for example, images can be dim or bright, close up or far away, large or small, and so on. Educating patients about submodalities of experience and teaching them that they can control these variables can be very helpful in reducing anxiety.

For example, we would like to suggest that you, the reader, think of something scary. Now, become aware of the scary image you are seeing that is associated with your fear. How close or far away from you is this projected image? Take a look. Now, move the image farther away from you, and as you do so, the image will probably get smaller. Be aware of your feelings about the picture as you use your brain in this way. Usually, fear or anxiety will diminish as you move the picture away and its image gets smaller.

Besides the submodalities of distance and size, another element of the visual system is brightness. Take a look at your scary picture again and brighten it increasingly as you pay attention to your feelings. Usually the act of brightening a scary picture until the details are washed out will decrease the fearful response.

Helping an anxious patient identify a key image that is associated with his or her fear and engaging in exercises similar to the one just described, especially when it is facilitated by trance, can be very productive. For example, one of us was recently consulted by a man suffering from persistent anxiety caused by witnessing a pedestrian being hit by a car and killed. The patient, Tom, stated that "the picture of the accident keeps staring me in the face." After hypnotic trance was induced, Tom was asked to imagine the picture that was so bothersome, and then to move it farther away, closer, and over to each side. When it was suggested that he move the picture far away from himself, Tom acknowledged that he felt better. Finally, it was suggested to Tom that he put the picture "way behind himself in the past where it belonged." The following suggestions were also made to Tom:

> "Tom, now you know what in some way you already knew. It's your brain and your images and your experiences, and *you can be in control, Tom* [embedded suggestion]. Just as you did here, *you can control your experience*, Tom, anytime you need to. And, since you did it here, you will find that more and more *you are in control* of all your experiences in comfortable ways."

A common cause of anxiety and confusion arises when a patient must make an important decision regarding two or more choices. Having the patient image the choices and then modulate submodalities of the images can generate an increased sense of control and facilitate decision making. For example, a patient who had a deadline about deciding on which of three job offers he was going to accept was familiarized during trance with visual submodalities and then told to vary these elements during self-hypnosis with an image or picture that represented each possible choice. He was told to see all three images at the same time, but to see each one differently with respect to how close or far, degree of brightness, location in his visual field, and so on, and to vary all these experiences. When he returned a week later he reported that the experience was very helpful to him and he had made his decision.

Similar submodality work can be facilitated for auditory and kinesthetic senses. For example, the next time a patient complains of anxiety and tells you that his "thoughts race in his mind and are too loud," tell him during trance to "be in control, and slow your inner voice down and lower it or make it softer." If the patient complains of difficulty doing this, simply tell him to "find the dials in your mind that control the speed and volume and turn them down." Hypnotic trance facilitates a patient's ability to learn increased control and helps patients to tap into their own creativity to accomplish what is necessary.

Existential therapists believe that the therapeutic goal is to reduce, not eliminate, anxiety. Patients must be helped to understand that some anxiety is a normal part of life. Often people who view themselves as fearful mistakeningly believe that others whom they see as healthier or more courageous than they never experience anxiety. As we stated earlier, part of psychotherapy is education, particularly education about what is normal in life. Patients must be taught that everyone experiences anxiety, and that healthy persons move ahead despite it and unhealthy ones run away from the situations that call forth the anxiety.

NORMAL ANXIETY

We offer one last note about the normal anxiety of life. Life is anxiety producing because almost all of the important things that happen to us have vague, mixed, and uncertain outcomes. Life comes with no guarantees. Even if the person you love loves you and is faithful to you, he or she could be hit by a bus tomorrow. Denial is a common mechanism many people use to control anxiety. Lovers do leave and we often struggle when we have to deal with behavior that suggests that those we labeled as all-good (friends, priests, politicians, and so on) are not *all*-good (or *all*-anything). Patients must learn to understand and accept life's lack of clarity and life's anxiety and not use denial as an antianxiety device.

CHAPTER 6

The Personal Meaning
of Symptoms

Some problems or symptoms can be dealt with briefly and strategically. Self-hypnosis can diminish anxiety and the use of power anchors can help a patient to conquer a simple phobia. However, many problems are so entrenched that they are resistant to change. It is particularly at these times that many clinicians will mistakenly dig in, draw up battle plans, and view a problem or symptoms as a pathology or as a disease that requires eradication. Conversely, an existentialist respects the reality that symptoms are meaningful within a particular patient's phenomenological world. An existentially oriented clinician therefore strives to understand the personal meanings of symptoms and takes this meaning into account while communicating and exploring with the patient. To promote change or a letting go of symptoms, an existentially oriented hypnotherapist helps the patient to explore and manifest potentials for healthier alternative patterns that will make meaningful sense within that patient's world. The communication of respect for symptoms and the process of exploring healthy alternative behaviors is usually enhanced by the use of hypnosis.

RELABELING SYMPTOMS

Looking at symptoms as meaningful and important signs constitutes a relabeling of symptoms. Such a framework is usually a new and refreshing one, not only to clinicians who have not yet embraced it in their work, but also to patients who have been told that their symptoms are crazy and meaningless.

To illustrate the importance of addressing the personal meanings of a problem in order to promote healthier change, let us take a look at students who complete most of the requirements for a doctoral degree but who cannot bring themselves to finish their dissertations. A surprising percentage of students entering Ph.D. programs seem to end up in this dilemma (known as "all but dissertation," or ABD) and many seek clinical intervention to help them get "unblocked." It would be nice if these people could simply respond to commonsense pleas, to time-management strategies, to behavior modification, or to self-incentive techniques, but usually this is not the case. Structured or programmed frameworks that do not account for the existential realities of the person are doomed. But when the personal meaning of blocking in regard to the dissertation is addressed, the chance of healthy progress increases.

The variety of possible reasons why a person does not complete his or her dissertation in order to get a Ph.D. speaks to the necessity of attending to a person's unique existence in the world. Our own experience with such cases indicates that inability to write a dissertation includes a wide spectrum of personality disorders. To one person, getting a Ph.D. meant leaving the playful world of youth and entering the hurtful adult world. To another person, getting a Ph.D. represented a weak capitulation to authoritarian demands. One student viewed her dissertation as having to be a masterpiece of perfection and therefore wrote, rewrote, and polished every paragraph; it was not long before she dreaded the entire project and viewed it as something to avoid. Another student was unaware of his fear that getting a Ph.D. would mean he would no longer fit within his family because no one else in his large family had even gone to college. One man we know resisted getting his Ph.D. because he unconsciously feared that something absolutely horrible would happen if he was very successful at accomplishing anything; his fear was associated with childhood trauma caused when his father was accidentally killed just after he was selected to assume an esteemed professional career position. Patients often will not be fully aware or even vaguely conscious of the personal meanings of their problem or symptoms. Hypnosis, which seems to facilitate inner awareness, is a helpful tool to help patients and clinicians understand the clinical problem within the context of the patient's world.

Arguing or fighting with patients is ineffective. Indeed, the therapist should never argue or fight with symptoms. Instead, the therapist should communicate respect that symptoms are existentially meaningful and important to the patient, and do this immediately and consistently. By so doing, the therapist "lays down his or her dukes" and helps to make the patient less inclined to fight and more inclined to be open to communication and further exploration. Such communication tends to immediately defuse resistance.

Instead of fighting with the patient or with his or her symptoms, we ally ourselves with the patient's resistance, thereby eliminating it. Since we sometimes define hypnosis simply as influential patterns of communication, the very act of communicating respect for symptoms can be considered a powerful hypnotic pattern or an example of what we call "little-*h* hypnosis," that is, hypnosis without a formal trance induction.

THE CASE OF SALLY

We were recently consulted for the first time by a seriously anorexic woman in her early 20s. Her family, friends, doctors, and psychotherapists had long been pleading with her to eat. When she came into our office she looked weak and sad, but she also displayed a defiant gleam in her eyes.

After a polite greeting, the therapist (C. M. C.) said:

"Sally, you're starving yourself and you're apparently doing a good job. I know people are concerned and maybe you are too. But I want you to know that I'm not going to fight or argue with you like the others. You obviously are quite powerful to be doing this to yourself. And you obviously have your own damn good reasons for doing it. I don't know what those reasons are; maybe you know or maybe you don't. But I'm here to talk to you about it if you choose to, and I'll be respectful about it. I know it's your life and your choices."

With that, Sally looked me straight in the eye to see if I was serious and saw that I was. She then agreed to talk. She soon revealed that she did not really know or understand herself why she was anorexic; all she knew was that it felt very important to her to be that way. Making no agreements to try to change, she did agree to be hypnotized in order to discover what her anorexia meant to her, what it did for her or how it helped her out in her world, and what healthier options she could engage in that would take care of her needs.

Sally came to hypnotherapy twice weekly for 6 months and then weekly for another 16 months. Hypnosis helped to reveal that Sally's anorexia, earlier in its development, had made her feel more in control amid parents who for years had been embroiled in a very conflicted marriage. Sally was not able to control her father's womanizing or end her parents' terrible arguments, but she could control what went into her body by starving herself, and she could control her parents by making them focus on her and her troubling illness. Then, as time went on, Sally's anorexia became meaningful as an identity for her. In and of itself, it became a way of life, of being-in-the-world. Controlling her weight became her constant preoccupation. Psychotherapy and support groups, medical appointments, and other pursuits related to her illness consumed much of Sally's time. Because of her illness, Sally worked only part time, continued to live at home, and was mostly supported by her parents.

In other words, her illness "helped" Sally to avoid "growing up." Sally's illness helped her to avoid the scary world of her own sexuality, taking responsibility for herself, and the adult world of commitment. As a result of her father's affairs and her parents' conflict, Sally perceived the adult world as a place filled with pain.

As these realities and meanings started to emerge, Sally's hypnotherapist helped her parents get into marital counseling. In this way Sally was relieved of her self-imposed role as the "sick" child whose illness kept her parents together. The therapist helped Sally to see other ways of being-in-the-world besides being "sick." Sally was encouraged to take risks, to socialize, and to date. She started college, and slowly she became more comfortable with herself, with other people, with other roles she could assume in the world, and with exploring her potentials. While this healthy, positive movement was taking place, Sally's anorexia seemed to fade away, and she slowly put on weight. Interestingly, one day Sally began the therapeutic session by announcing, "I've decided not to be anorexic anymore." When she was asked to explain this decision, Sally stated, "I really can't explain this to you, other than to say that I'm just choosing now to be a normal person like other people." That choice by Sally signaled the end to her illness. We have heard other patients making such statements, taking positive positions, and asserting their choice of being-in-the-world; such transformations buttress our decision to embrace an existential framework when dealing with human behavior and change.

THE CASE OF JAN

To further illustrate the importance of understanding and respecting the personal meanings of symptoms, we will now present another detailed case study. This case also points out the role of hypnosis in uncovering the existential meanings of problems and in facilitating the patient's generation of healthy new patterns and increased personal power.

Jan was 44 years old, had been married 17 years, and wanted to lose about 65 pounds. Jan was about 5 feet, 3 inches, in height and weighed 185 pounds. Jan's weight prior to marriage had been about 120 pounds. Members of her family of origin all had relatively normal weights. Jan had tried numerous diets and dietary programs and usually had been able to lose about 25 pounds. However, she told us that "as soon as I start to look good, I screw up, and soon the weight returns." She stated that like her weight, her marriage to Tom had its ups and downs, and that her husband complained about her weight, which she resented. Jan worked as an insurance underwriter; her husband owned a successful printing company.

Jan was frustrated and felt very stuck about her weight. She chose her therapist because of his reputation for doing hypnosis, and she hoped that hypnosis could help her.

Jan said that her husband wanted the therapist to let him know what he could do to help. The therapist sent Tom a note, shared with Jan, which read as follows:

> Dear Mr. Smith:
> Thank you for your kind offer to help your wife out. Since Jan is very enthusiastic about dieting, and since I'm sure you'd like her to be healthy, what you can do is make sure she doesn't diet too much or lose weight too quickly. Therefore, would you please remind her, at least three or four times a week, not to overdo it with her dieting and not to lose too much weight too quickly.

This paradoxical directive to the husband was based on the evidence presented by Jan of her resentment of, and resistance to, her husband's complaints about her weight, and the likelihood that she would resist any strong suggestion or push by her husband. The directive was a form of "symptom prescription" technique (Zeig, 1980a, 1980b; Haley, 1984; Seltzer, 1986). As far as Jan was concerned, she was told not to lose too much weight too quickly. This was aimed at channeling the energy of her resistance in a healthy direction and toward her therapeutic objective.

The therapist hypnotized Jan at her second session. It was obvious to the therapist that merely offering simple suggestions to diet and exercise would not suffice for her to lose and keep off weight. As is almost always the case with symptoms or patterns that will not budge, *the personal meaning of symptoms must be addressed before change can be expected to occur.*

Here is a transcript of the interesting dialogue that ensued between the therapist and Jan while she experienced her trance.

THERAPIST: Jan, I want to be respectful about this, so I'm not just going to suggest you lose 65 pounds. We need to understand what this weight means to you. You've tried to lose that weight many times before, you manage to lose about half of it, and then you powerfully call it quits. So I'd like to suggest, Jan, that you take some time now and explore what weighing 185 pounds means to you and also what it means to you to lose 65 pounds. Take the time you need in the next minute or two and please nod your head when you have done this good work.

[A few moments later, Jan nodded her head.]

JAN: Weighing 185 pounds to me is disgusting—the way it looks, and how unhealthy it is. Losing those 65 pounds means depriving myself of eating lots of things I like to eat. And it means lots of hard work to accomplish this.

THERAPIST: Okay, those things are important, but I have a feeling that there's more to all this. Take your time now, Jan, and let go in your mind and become aware of other meanings or associations that weighing 185 pounds or losing the excess weight has for you. How does the weight help you, Jan? What do you get from it that you desire or need? What does it help you to avoid that you don't want or that you fear? Most important, Jan, what would you lose if you gave up the weight?

JAN: The idea of losing that weight makes me furious. It's Tom and his complaints about how I look. I don't want to give into him.

THERAPIST: It sounds like holding onto the weight is a way of feeling in control and powerful in your marriage. Well, what other ways can you feel powerful with Tom so you can feel free enough to lose the weight? It's likely that there are healthier alternatives than being overweight. Take a minute or two and go into your mind and come up with some other healthier patterns or ways to be with Tom that will provide you with the control and power that you need.

[After some inner exploration and some help from the therapist Jan decided that she would start asserting herself more with her husband, now that she knew that the therapist would be available for support.]

THERAPIST: So far, Jan, you've decided to start being more assertive with Tom and that will help you to feel enough control and power in the relationship to free you up to diet and not feel like you're giving in. First, you've decided that you won't go to his mother's every Sunday with him, but rather only occasionally. Second, next Fall, no more of that dreaded bowling league for you. Are there any other things that come to mind or that you experience when you think about losing the excess weight and weighing 120 pounds?

JAN: It scares me.

THERAPIST: What about it scares you, Jan?

JAN: I'm not sure. I just feel anxious when I see myself at 120 pounds.

THERAPIST: Well, take a look again at yourself, and then be open to anything else that might occur to you, Jan. There's something about looking like that that's making you anxious. Is there anything else that you see, or hear, or feel as you imagine this?

JAN: Yes. I see a door.

[At this point Jan realized that the door she saw in her mind was her own front door. She then became aware that she was afraid that if she dieted down to her previous 120 pounds, she might feel more confident and brave enough to leave her marriage with the hope of finding a more fulfilling relationship. She also became aware of the likelihood that her being at a more attractive weight increased the chances of other men flirting with her. This did not scare her as much as her fear that she might say yes to a flirtatious advance.]

THERAPIST: Jan, it's likely that losing that weight will open up all kinds of doors for you. But you will always have a choice to go through a door or not. Actually, most, if not all, of these choices, like staying in your marriage or having an affair, have been available to you all along, but you just didn't know that. Perhaps your weight has been a way of avoiding all these choices and all this freedom. Choices and freedom can make many people anxious; and instead of dealing with all these potentials, many people just avoid the choices. But let's face it, Jan, you haven't been that happy anyway; so you might have nothing to lose by losing the weight, except the wait to lose the weight. And when you lose the weight, Jan, then you'll gain in other healthy, powerful ways; for example, you'll feel good about the way you look and about the compliments you'll likely get from others. And perhaps, most importantly, even though you might feel a little anxious with the realization of all the choices available to you, knowing that you have all kinds of choices is very freeing and feels powerful. So you have a choice now, Jan, to diet and exercise and lose the weight, and with that choice you may feel anxious or maybe that feeling is really very exciting about the choices and potentials that await you on this journey. Or you can choose to just avoid the whole thing altogether, as you've chosen in the past. This is an important choice for you. That's why, this week, I'd like you to continue to do self-hypnosis knowing that the objective is for you to powerfully make the best choice for yourself, Jan.

[At this point, the therapist suggested that Jan alert soon from her trance and the session ended.]

The hypnotic session just described illustrates some important aspects of existential hypnotherapy. First, trance was utilized to facilitate Jan's awareness of the personal or existential meanings of her weight gain and her past difficulties in dieting. Notice the respect communicated by the therapist about the symptoms and their importance to the patient. In contrast to arguing or fighting, such communication defuses resistance, allowing a freer exploration of the issues involved. Notice also that throughout the dialogue the therapist takes every opportunity to frame things positively and to communicate the positive message that Jan has choices, power, and control available to her. For example, he tells her that she has "powerfully" called it quits each time she has lost about half her excess weight and that she has been powerful in not giving in to her husband's complaints about her weight. To reinforce the idea that she is in control, the therapist also allows Jan to do most of the important work herself. Allowing the patient to do the work is more empowering. Finally, to indicate his respect for the reality of her choices and power, the therapist directs Jan to take a week to choose either to continue to hold onto the weight or to utilize other, presumably more healthy, patterns. Sometimes, under these circumstances, a patient will choose to continue with the status quo and keep her or his symptoms. However, it is our experience that even when that choice is made, the patient feels better about herself or himself and generally more powerful, a changed attitude that displays itself in other healthy ways.

Notice that the therapist did not stop or accept Jan's first response about what the weight or losing it meant to her (that it was "disgusting," and that losing the weight meant "depriving" herself). In existential hypnotherapy it is important to keep in mind that *all important meanings, conscious and unconscious, of the presenting problem or symptoms need to be addressed.*

IDENTIFYING PERSONAL MEANING

Quite often a patient is not aware or at least consciously aware of important meanings of his or her problematic patterns. Hypnosis can facilitate such awareness. Often the therapist's help is also needed. In Jan's case, the therapist asked a series of questions (How does the weight help you, Jan? What do you get from it that you desire or need? and so on) intended to help Jan with her search for the existential meaning of her symptoms. A more complete list of such exploratory questions is presented in Table 1.

Another strategy that can help a patient to identify the personal meaning or importance of symptoms is to present a multiple-choice array of possible meanings that might be associated with the patient's symptoms. The choices should include possible meanings based on the therapist's perceptions and intuitions about the patient as well as meanings gleaned from past clinical experiences with similar patients. When using this technique we like to present these possibilities by talking about other patients we have treated who had similar symptoms and what these patients discovered in terms of the meaning to them of the symptoms. Watch for subtle non-

TABLE 1. Questions That Facilitate Awareness of Personal Meanings of Symptoms (X)

1. What does X mean to you?
2. What does it mean to you to be without X?
3. How does X help you out or what payoffs or benefits do you get from X?
4. How does X give you more power or control?
5. How does X help you to feel safe?
6. What does X help you to avoid?
7. How does X get you more attention or love?
8. What does X help you to express?
9. What was it like for you before X?
10. What was going on in your life when X appeared?
11. How did things change after there was X?
12. What will happen when there is no X?
13. After X disappears, what will your life be like 1 year (5 years, 10 years, 20 years) later?
14. Who else ever had X or has it now?
15. Assume there is an inner part of you responsible for X or associated with X:
    - What does that part of you look like?
    - What color is that part of you?
    - What does that part of you sound like or what does it have to say about X?
    - What does that part of you feel like?

verbal cues from patients as you do this to gather information about them. This process is only helpful if the hypnotherapist has experience and knowledge about a patient's
specific symptoms.

If a patient still has difficulty consciously offering inter-
pretations of the meaning of his or her symptoms, we may
turn to ideomotor signaling techniques (for example, hypnoti-
cally setting up and using finger singles for "Yes" and "No")
to help identify important meanings. We look for minimal or
unconscious cues (for example, a slight head nod for "Yes")
to help confirm the validity of what a patient reports to us or
to help identify important meanings of symptoms not conscious to the patient. When we present a multiple-choice array
of possibilities to a patient, we will "zero in" on a choice that
the patient seemed to react to with positive minimal cues.

All these strategies can help the patient and the therapist to identify the personal meanings of symptoms. They can
also be employed to help the patient generate healthy patterns to substitute for his or her symptoms. For example, a
multiple-choice array of healthier alternatives can be presented to the patient for consideration and ideomotor signaling or observation of minimal cues can be utilized to confirm
the appropriateness or "fit," consciously and unconsciously,
of a healthier alternative for a particular patient.

Hypnosis helps patients to become aware of the unconscious meanings of their symptoms. By its very nature of
increasing openness regarding imagination and potentials,
hypnosis or trance also facilitates patients identifying and
using new patterns of experience, perceptions, or realities, and
new patterns of behavior that are healthier for the patient.
For example, Jan realized that she could assert herself in
healthier ways with her husband instead of being overweight.
She also realized that losing weight would "open doors" for
her, that she would have the choice to go through a door or
not, and that exploring these choices could be exciting and
powerful.

The communication employed by the therapist with Jan
includes some interesting hypnotic patterns. First, the patient's
language usage was paced and utilized throughout the ses-

sion. For example, when Jan stated that she felt anxious "When I *see* myself at 120 pounds," the therapist asked her to "Take a look again" at what might be causing this anxiety. Also, the therapist utilized Jan's image of a door to suggest to her the existential notion that "all kinds of doors" were available to her because of existential freedom and choice.

The transcript of this hypnotic session also reveals the use of confusion (Erickson & Rossi, 1976a, 1979) when the therapist suggests to Jan that she has "nothing to lose by losing the weight, except the wait to lose the weight." Verbal confusion like this tends to decrease conscious analysis and resistance and to increase suggestibility. The next statement in the transcript, "And when you lose the weight, Jan, then you'll gain in other healthy, powerful ways," illustrates use of the "apposition of opposites" described by Erickson and Rossi (1976a, 1979). They described how the natural tendency of people to balance out opposites or to achieve homeostasis can be utilized toward therapeutic ends. The interspersal technique (Erickson & Rossi, 1976a, 1979) or embedded suggestions (Grinder & Bandler, 1981) were also used by the therapist by subtly changing voice tone on key phrases and/ or by pausing slightly just before and after a suggestion. For example, the suggestions to "lose that weight, Jan," were often communicated and the suggestion to "powerfully make the best choice for yourself, Jan," appears at the very end of the hypnotic session. Finally, the typically existential tendency to relabel anxiety as excitement is illustrated when the therapist states to Jan that she "may feel anxious or maybe that feeling is really very exciting about the choices and potentials that await you on this journey."

Jan chose to diet and lose weight. In ensuing hypnotic sessions other meanings and potentials of hers, avoided by her past pattern of excess weight, were addressed. During hypnotic sessions she was told some metaphorical stories, such as the Ogre Story (see Chapter 9), and these helped to support her journey to increased personal power. Mental rehearsal and power anchors were also used to help Jan. For example, after she lost about 30 pounds and began to get many compliments and increased attention from people, a power anchor was used during trance as Jan imagined dealing powerfully with an attractive man who was acting seductively toward her. This mental rehearsal and use of the power anchor helped her to address one of the fears that she had about the weight loss.

Jan's husband was delighted about her weight loss but unhappy about the personal power she displayed, which he resisted. She succeeded in losing and keeping off the weight and the couple ended up in marital counseling.

Existential Therapy's Metaphors

In the everyday life-world much of the time our patients experience their lives and interpret those lives by means of symbols and metaphors. When someone says "My heart is heavy," no one reaches for a scale to measure his or her pathology. When someone states "I'm feeling blue," the therapist does not remark that his or her skin tone looks normal. Yet too often as "professionals" and "scientists" we forget about the world of metaphors and get stuck communicating only in literal, left brain language. We have found that sometimes it is more effective to make a simple metaphorical statement such as "The ball's in your court" rather than give a long lecture on the need to take personal responsibility.

This is especially true with regard to hypnotic communication because when the language of hypnotherapy keeps pace with the symbolic and metaphoric realities of the patient, rapid healing can often be facilitated. This can happen even when the therapist does not understand exactly the how or the why of the therapeutic result. We will start this discussion about metaphors with the notion of the unconscious. The unconscious is a metaphor imprinted into the *Lebenswelt's* (life-world) understanding of the human being from the psychoanalytic fable. This is a metaphor we use with every hypnotherapy patient and no one has ever questioned its existence. We use it because it provides an excellent excuse or explanation for change. Why do people need an excuse for change? Often they have been stuck in a psychological "rut" or have exhibited a negative pattern of behavior for a long time. Their inability to get out of this rut, to end the negative behavior, frustrates them and all who care for them. If patients entered therapy and all of a sudden freed themselves from the rut or reformed their behavior too quickly they might become anxious about the speed of their transformation. They would fear, and rightly so, that a rapid reformation would leave them open to the charge that they could have changed much sooner. If, on the other hand, they can argue that the change occurred because a professional intervened in their mysterious unconscious processes, then the change can be accepted without the burden of acknowledging that their past behaviors were always under their own control.

The unconscious is vague and metaphoric, yet existentially real, to most patients. During an initial trance session we usually introduce the concept of the unconscious casually:

> "The nice thing about trance is that there is nothing that you have to do. You don't even need to pay attention when I am speaking to you. That is because I am speaking to your unconscious mind and I know that your unconscious will be listening, so the rest of you can drift away if you want. Now when I say this to people they often ask, 'Dr. King, what do you mean by the unconscious mind?,' but you know and I know and that's okay."

Patients never question what this means. They are left with an illusion that we have had a discussion about the unconscious and have come to an agreement as to its meaning. As therapists, we do not care what the patient's actual beliefs are concerning this metaphor. What is important to us is the knowledge that each patient uses it in his or her own way in the hypnotherapy work.

Different kinds of metaphors are used in existential hypnotherapy. Later in this chapter we will detail the use of metaphoric stories for therapeutic gains. One of the most frequently used and useful classes of metaphors is visual imagery. This is also an area where there is a clear distinction between the work of an existentially oriented therapist and other kinds of therapists. Almost all hypnotherapists use visual imagery in their treatment designs. Most use a type of guided imagery; that is, the therapist helps develop all or part of the imagery. In existential hypnotherapy all of the imagery comes from the patient. More often than not, the patient produces metaphoric rather than literal imagery.

METAPHORIC IMAGES FOR PAIN CONTROL

To illustrate our methods, we will give examples from our work with patients who entered hypnotherapy for help with chronic physical pain, and then we will discuss using metaphoric visual imagery to help patients deal with strong emotional experiences. When we work with pain patients, while they are in trance, we ask them to take an imaginary trip inside their bodies to the location of the discomfort to see what it looks like. Even patients who initially have difficulty getting a clear image will usually be able to produce one after a few trance sessions. When the patient reports what he or she sees, we next ask the patient what he or she thinks will improve the situation. Sometimes patients insist that they do not know; with such patients, we offer several alternatives, and ask the patient to choose among them. We always encourage our patients not to worry about "reality." We say that we do not care what the pain or damage really looks like inside of them. We tell them that we want to work with whatever their experience is. The same holds true for the solution. This process will come into sharper focus with the aid of some examples.

> A 55-year-old salesman came into therapy complaining of severe ankle pain that prevented him from working more than half a day at a time. This pain had been getting worse for about 5 years. He reported that three different doctors had been unable to help him. In trance, he was asked to imagine what the pain looked like. He said it looked like a school of piranhas were attacking him and he could see the teeth literally penetrating his skin. When he was asked what he thought would be helpful to the

situation, he was unable to come up with an answer. The therapist suggested to him that while in trance he imagine a group of men and women in dental outfits carrying soft, rubber caps for the piranhas' teeth. He was then asked to imagine that as these piranhas came toward him the caps were placed on their teeth. This exercise was repeated three times in the therapist's office and he was asked to do this as a self-hypnosis homework assignment nightly for 3 weeks. By the end of the third week he reported only mild irritations where the disabling pain used to be. As he left therapy for the last time he was cautioned to be careful while he was driving since the tickling of the piranhas with the caps on their teeth might be distracting to him.

A 40-year-old woman was referred by an oral surgeon for temporomandibular joint pain and spasms that did not respond to surgery. On intake, it was discovered that the woman had many emotional problems, especially a bad marriage. She stayed in therapy for approximately 9 months to work on these issues. Near the beginning of the therapy she was asked in trance to take an imaginary trip inside her jaw and to note what she experienced on that trip. She reported that she saw images that reminded her of the pegs of guitar strings and they seemed to be wound too tight. For the next 2 months during trance, and as a self-hypnosis assignment, she was asked to take a trip inside her jaw and to loosen one of the two pegs, alternating sides of the mouth just a fraction of an inch each time. After years of pain and spasms she reported an almost total reduction in that pain and absence of spasms. The spasms and pain stayed in remission as long as this patient did self-hypnosis 3 to 4 times a week using this imagery. When she did not do self-hypnosis for about a month the pain returned and it took another couple of weeks of hypnosis using visual imagery before she felt good again. This process has kept her pain-free for about 4 years except for the "booster shots" she needs about every 9 months when she gets careless about doing her self-hypnosis.

A very attractive 30-year-old professional was referred to therapy by her physician for help with severe spasms of the esophagus and related pain. She had just completed an 8-day hospital stay during which intense diagnostic tests revealed no physical problems. She had been complaining of pain for about 2 years and said that it seemed to be getting worse. During intake, no psychological stressors could be identified. The woman had a healthy childhood background, was in a satisfying long-term relationship, and had a career that was moving ahead in an orderly, planned direction. During trance she was asked to take an imaginery trip inside herself. She reported that she saw an iceball with thousands of horns on the outside that was located right in the middle of her chest. When asked what would help the situation, she replied that if she could attack the iceball with an icepick it would be reduced in size. She also asked that her boyfriend help her to do this work. After four sessions spread out over 6 weeks and related self-hypnosis at home she reported for the first time in years that she was spasm- and pain-free. This case was followed up and there was no reported pain for the first year. The entire treatment for this case consisted of the imagery work. There was no associated psychotherapy.

A 20-year-old woman reported numbness in one or both of her legs whenever she got nervous. The nervousness appeared in response to social situations and school performance demands. In trance, she took a trip inside her legs and noticed that her nerve endings were covered with a white plastic wrapping. Within about 4 weeks she learned that whenever she got tense and began to experience a numbness that she could take an imaginary trip with some sorority sisters and unwrap the plastic from the nerves.

As strange as it may seem to psychotherapists who have never used this type of imagery, all the patients described here and hundreds more have entered hypnotherapy with long-term chronic pain and showed significant relief in just a matter of weeks using the imagery solutions that made sense to them. To repeat, we attempt to do as little guiding as possible; however, some patients do need our encouragement, especially in coming up with solutions associated with the original images that they experience.

DEALING WITH DISTURBING FEELINGS

There are many of ways to deal with feelings in psychotherapy and hypnotherapy. One of the fastest, most effective ways to modify feelings that are disturbing to patients is to utilize metaphoric visual images of the feelings that are produced by the patient. Some of what we will present below is a modification of the work of David Grove (1989).

When a patient wants to modify a disturbing feeling, we will ask that patient during trance to notice where in the body he or she feels that feeling. When the patient identifies the place, we then ask, "The feelings feel like a what?" Usually this one question is enough to encourage the patient to imagine his or her feeling as an object. If not, we encourage image production by asking questions such as What is its shape? What is its size? What is its color? Once the patient fixes an image, we next ask, "What would that object like to have happen?" and "Can it happen?" We then encourage the patient during the hypnotherapy in the office and at home during self-hypnosis to allow the image to develop in a way that the object would like. Again, examples will help to clarify this process:

> A 28-year-old woman entered therapy complaining of severe anxiety associated with sexual relations with her husband. She claimed to be in love with her husband, and said that the relationship was good in every other way and that she even felt sexually attracted to him. She could not understand her symptoms. In taking a family history the therapist learned that the patient's grandfather lived with her for the first 7 years of her life and that he was an abusive alcoholic. A few years previously, the father had told his daughter that she had probably been sexually abused by this grandfather. There had been a mysterious accident that the patient could not remember; her hips were broken when she was 3 years old and only her grandfather was home with her at the time of the accident. In trance, during the third hypnotic session, she was asked what the anxiety felt like and described it as a big, black bowling ball. She was asked where this bowling ball was located and she answered, "In my groin area." She was then asked what the black bowling ball wanted to have happen. She said that the black bowling ball wanted to get in a red wagon. She was asked, "Can the bowling ball get in the red wagon?" She said, "Yes." She then imaged the black bowling ball jumping into a little red wagon that traveled down a bumpy road to the edge of a

cliff, where the wagon overturned and the bowling ball fell over the cliff. The patient described being able to see the bowling ball shattering in many pieces at the bottom of the large cliff. The next week the patient reported having sex with her husband without any associated anxiety for the first time in a few years. The patient remembered many happy childhood moments with her older brother pulling her around in a red wagon and believed the problem was associated with the red wagon. She had no idea of the meaning of the black ball.

A 40-year-old woman entered therapy complaining of severe social isolation and resulting depression. After a few sessions it became clear that the predominant feeling this patient was experiencing was anger. She had the insight to recognize that she herself would not want to be the friend of someone who was so chronically angry as she was. In trance, she was asked to imagine what the anger looked like and she said it was like a knife in her heart. She was asked what the knife wanted to do, and she answered that the knife wanted to cut off fingers. She was asked, "Can the knife cut off fingers?" She replied, "Yes." Then, without direction from the therapist, she imagined hands (without an attached face or body) and she cut off the fingers. When she did that she smiled and said, "Now they can't touch me anymore." This was the first insight she had into her own history of being a sexually abused child. It was also the beginning of therapeutic gains for this patient.

A 40-year-old man entered therapy. He seemed to be a perfect match for the patient discussed above. He complained that he had no friends at work and no history of intimate relationships except for a short marriage that had ended 4 years earlier. He described himself as a very angry fellow. During hypnosis he was asked to imagine his anger and he said it was like a big volcano spouting out all kinds of lava. He was asked where this big volcano was located and he said, "Right in the middle of my heart." He was then asked what this big volcano wanted to do, and he replied that it wanted to squirt hot lava all over everybody else. When asked if it *could* squirt hot lava all over everybody else, he said, "No, because I would feel too guilty." He was then asked to imagine what the guilt was like. He said it was big slushy volume of water like a water balloon. He was asked where this big slushy body of water was located and he said, "In my stomach." The therapist then asked, "Can this big volcano with the hot lava go to this big slushy water balloon?" He answered, "No." The therapist then said, "Can the big slushy body of water like a water balloon go to the volcano?" He smiled and said, "Yes." He then described an imaginary experience of a water balloon as big as a planet drenching the volcano and putting it out. This experience was repeated three times in sessions with the therapist and daily for a month during self-hypnosis. The patient reported significant reductions in his feelings of anger and was able to begin to move forward in his life by establishing healthy social relationships.

A 55-year-old female had been in therapy for 6 months talking about an unpleasant childhood and trying to resolve some issues concerning her parents. She also was discussing job problems and issues about social relationships. She was also using hypnosis for pain management after an automobile accident. After some brief success with the therapy, the process reached an impasse and the patient started to feel ashamed about "blocking and not moving on." In trance she was asked what the block was like and she imagined a large oak tree. When asked where it was lodged, she said it was in her head and it would not let anything pass. When she was asked what had to happen or what did the large oak tree want to happen, she said it felt ashamed because it would not let anything get through. She was asked to imagine what her shame was like and she saw it as a vague object in her right arm. A session later she was able to imagine the object in her right arm as a pickax and over the next 3 weeks she used that pickax to chop the large oak tree into small pieces. Within a month therapy seemed to move forward faster than before.

GUIDED METAPHORIC IMAGES

As we mentioned earlier, we try to let our patients generate their own images. Such images have a personal meaning to them, even though we or they themselves may not consciously understand this meaning. Occasionally we do use some forms of guided imagery in our work. In these cases we strive to allow as much ambiguity and openness as possible to leave each patient with plenty of freedom to fill in the gaps with their own personal details and images.

We commonly begin trance with a formal introduction that in part asks patients to go into their mind to a favorite place or just to visit someplace they would like to be as we talk to them. We give the patient permission not to stay in this favorite place for the entire trance experience, but the very act of directing the person to this type of place is a guided experience. Unlike most other hypnotherapists we have observed or read about, we do not direct patients to a specific place, such as a beach, or even ask them ahead of time where they want to go. There are two reasons for this. First, if we know where they are going it is easy to mismatch experiences. We may know that a patient is going to a beach. If I have just returned from Jamaica, I may start describing its white sand beaches and clear, green water. But the patient may have taken himself or herself to Atlantic City which has not had white beaches or clear water since 1952. Thus my words will be out of sync with the patient's experience. Second, when patients go into trance and let go of conscious control they often take themselves to places they would have never imagined in a pretrance discussion. Often patients find themselves at their grandparents' house or someplace else they have not been to in 30 years. The places patients choose to visit can by themselves lead to therapeutic insights.

At times we tell our patients something like this: "In your unconscious there are all sorts of components and tools. There are dials, switches, levers, buttons, valves of all kinds. Whatever you might need to turn one thing up or on, or to turn something else down or off exists in your unconscious. In your inner mind you might wonder just how helpful all these resources will be for you."

Similarly, to help patients gain increased control over a feeling, a sensation, or bodily pain, we might utilize the following image:

"In the back of your mind is a huge control room, just like you might see in a nuclear power plant—like the one you may have seen in the movie *The China Syndrome*. And in that control room there are many panels with dials, switches, levers, and buttons. Please nod your head when you image this control room in your mind. Good. Now, I'd like to suggest that you find the particular dial, switch, or button that controls that angry feeling and nod your head when you see it." [We then direct the patient to use this image to modify the feeling in question.]

THERAPEUTIC STORIES AS METAPHORS

Stories are part of every patient's life. In fact, all cultures have used stories to disseminate knowledge and pass along traditions, moral values, and laws. Since existential therapy is at its best when in harmony with the patient's life-world, it stands to reason that storytelling will play a major role in existential hypnotherapy.

There are a number of advantages to using metaphoric stories in hypnotherapy. First, these metaphors produce data that are both visual and auditory. If the story is well told, the patient who is in trance will experience visual representations stimulated by the story. The details of the story should be left somewhat vague so that these visual images are a product of the patient's personal meaning system; in other words, the images are influenced by, but not dictated by, the story. All the advantages of using visual imagery that were previously discussed in this chapter also apply to the use of storytelling. In addition, the stories carry within them therapeutic language that the patient hears from the therapist.

A second advantage of stories is that they can be used as an indirect form of communication that has therapeutic advantages we have detailed elsewhere (King et al., 1983; Citrenbaum et al., 1985). To summarize the main advantage, the symptoms patients came into therapy to "get rid of" always have a personal meaning for them (see Chapter 6) and often continue to have a secondary gain associated with them. For example, the cigarettes a patient smokes may "connect" him or her to a deceased parent who smoked the same brand, or a physical illness may help a patient avoid certain responsibilities. Thus patients are often resistant to the very changes they consciously desire so much. Every therapist knows that with most patients therapy is like a boxing match: when the session begins the gloves go up. If, however, you can do therapy while you are appearing not to be doing therapy— for example, if you tell a seemingly casual story about a friend—then the patient has no reason to be resistant. The therapist almost never hears the phrase, "Yes, but" following a story.

Many times we are asked, "Don't patients resent it when you take up their therapy time with your personal stories?" Never. Patients are complimented that you think enough about them as people to share something about yourself. We also believe that patients intuitively understand that these stories contain messages intended for them.

A third advantage of storytelling as a hypnotherapeutic technique is that most patients really enjoy listening to stories. Therapeutic stories that are indirect or covert in terms of the therapeutic messages they transmit are likely to be the most influential because they bypass the patient's conscious analysis and conscious or unconscious resistance. However, even when the meaning of a story is quite apparent, storytelling can still be more powerful therapeutically than directly telling the patient the "same old thing in the same old way." Phillip Barker (1985, p. vii) points out that "direct teaching of behavioral laws and principles often meets with resistance on the part of those being taught because the message is too direct, too personal, too shocking or, not infrequently, too difficult to understand." When a good therapeutic metaphor is constructed it becomes like a Zen *Koan*: you cannot see through it or use logical, lineral thinking to understand the message. It becomes a form of experiential learning.

Hypnosis and Storytelling

Communicating with patients through the use of metaphorical stories is effective even when you are not doing formal trance work. Many times we will tell a story before we begin the hypnotherapy, or at least that is the patient's perception. This does not mean that the patient is not in a trance when he or she hears the story. A story well told is in itself a hypnotic induction. It is a type of the informal or "little-*h* hypnosis" that we discussed at the beginning of this book. Most of the time, however, we like to deliver the metaphor after the patient has been hypnotized. There are three reasons why we believe the experience of trance enhances the therapeutic value of the story. First, the focused attention of trance enhances the production of all sensory experience and especially of visual images. In fact, there are many people who have such trouble experiencing visual imagery that it cannot be used as part of a trance induction, but who can experience imagery after they have been hypnotized. Second, the subject in trance is a less critical listener who is not particularly bothered by therapeutically purposeful gaps, vagueness, or sequences that may seem out of order to a different listener.

A third very important value of trance relative to therapeutic storytelling is that the process of hypnosis becomes a good excuse for telling the story. We often say something like this to our patients: "Now that you have achieved your trance, all that matters for a while is what your unconscious mind does. It doesn't even matter what I say. I talk just for the hypnotic patter, to be in touch with you. One of the things I like to talk about is _____." We then tell a metaphorical story or two. The term "hypnotic patter" does not really mean much to us, but it is a term most of the patients seem to feel they have heard before and it therefore seems legitimate to them. Now we have an excuse to talk about anything.

Elements in Therapeutic Stories

There are two basic elements in the stories we develop for our patients. First, many of our stories offer solutions, strategies, or new behaviors that we would like our patients to try. These are expressed in the words of the stories and/or the images produced by the patient. Thus the patient "experiences" the message, but often without consciously knowing that it comes from the therapist. The value of this process is that the patient himself or herself can take all the credit for positive change, which is very empowering. Remember the "let go" metaphors we discussed in Chapter 3. Often patients report within a few weeks after hearing these stories how they said to themselves, "Why don't you let go," or "Just let go," and then they tell us how they were able to change a habit or pattern of behavior. Of course, we never remind them of the story that put this idea in their minds.

A second element in many of our stories is an appeal to the patient's internal resources for problem solving. In some stories we will not communicate any direct strategy for change or indicate any new patterns, but we will metaphorically suggest that an unstated solution is available. When we first learned about this strategy we were skeptical about its value, but we have since discovered that this technique works. We cannot explain the process by which it works: we just know that it does work. We usually use a story about someone old and wise, or someone with authority to represent that part of the patient that can solve his or her own problems. Over the years we have seen a number of patients who show remarkable improvement after experiencing one of these stories, improvement that we cannot explain except by believing that their story stimulated an internal personal resource.

Examples of Therapeutic Stories

A number of books discuss how to develop stories and offer hundreds of examples (see Rosen, 1982; Lankton & Lankton, 1983; Barker, 1985; Bettelheim, 1977; Gordon, 1978; Wallis, 1985; Zeig, 1980c).

We will only give a few case examples here because we believe it is important that each therapist learn how to develop stories that reflect the patient–therapist dialectic that emerges idiosyncratically in each individual case. We have supervised too many professionals who tend to rely on stock stories they read in a textbook. After presenting these examples we will briefly discuss some principles of story-making for the existentially oriented hypnotherapist.

A 29-year-old African-American male was referred to us by a local hospital where he had been tested for severe head-aches. No physical abnormalities had been uncovered. During intake the man reported that the biggest stress in his life was sexual dysfunction. He was impotent most of the time he attempted to have sex and suffered from premature ejac-ulations on those few occasions when he was not impotent. He said his sexual problems had begun with the crib death of his child 2 years earlier. Within a year of that crib death he divorced his wife. As a single man he dated regularly but suffered embarrassment and stress due to his problem. The headaches started around the time of his divorce and had been getting increasingly worse. During the second session the therapist told him that he could be helped with his problem, but also told him that they would not work on the problem for a couple of weeks until the patient learned to do hypno-sis and self-hypnosis. While in trance, during this first hyp-notic session, the therapist told the patient the following story:

> "You know, on beautiful days like today I like to go white-water rafting down the Youghiogheny River at Ohiopyle State Park. Now I don't know if you know anything about that river but I learned something very interesting just a short while ago. Up until 10 years ago the river was wild and uncontrolled, totally at the mercy of the elements. Many times, like in the spring, the water rushed down too fast and people like me couldn't go on it. The majority of times, like most of the late summer, the water was much too low and people couldn't go on it much either. They decided to build a dam to control the river, so they went 10 miles up north to a town called Confluence. Now the terrain was very rocky so they had to call in a master engineer from Washington, D.C. He looked around for a

while and finally figured out what he had to do. Soon he was able to build the dam and now the water was *hardly* ever too low and *hardly* ever too rapid so that we couldn't have fun."

After this story the therapist changed the topic and did many of the things he would normally do during a first hypnotic session. The next week the patient came back and reported that he had had two different sexual experiences and that both were extremely satisfying. He was very surprised at this turn of events and asked the therapist if he had any idea why he seemed to be cured. The therapist said, "No, but we don't need to ask questions when things are going well." The man discontinued therapy, but returned about a year later for some help on different issues related to his work. At that later session he reported satisfying sexual experiences all the time during the year and mentioned he was now engaged. He later fathered two children and sent pictures of each to the therapist at Christmastime. The patient seemed to have a sense that the therapist had helped him with his sexual problem but he did not really know how; quite frankly, the therapist is not totally sure, either.

You will have noticed that all the elements in this story had to do with the patient's problem. The engineer had to go up north (the direction from the genital area to the mind or brain); the terrain was rocky and it was a tough thing to do; a master engineer (a metaphor for the unconcious mind or inner resources of the patient) had to be called in; and the words "hard" and "have fun" contain embedded psychosexual suggestions.

We have used the next two stories or variations thereof with a number of different patients. The patients reported that these stories particularly seemed to stimulate very interesting and clear visual imagery that seemed to be helpful to them in solving their problems.

"You know, _____ [patient's name], I just heard an interesting story from China. The patient walks up to a wiseman and says, 'I don't know what to do, I feel like there's a dog with his mouth around my leg pulling me to the East and another dog with his mouth around my leg pulling me to the West. What should I do, wiseman?' The wiseman looks at him and says, 'Just feed the dog if you want to win!'"

"I just came back from the western United States where I visited a modern, progressive zoo and had an interesting talk with an old zookeeper who had been there for many years. She told me that before they had this progressive zoo, when more traditional cages were used, she had a favorite animal whose cage was too small for it. She said all the animal did all day was pace back and forth 15 yards from one side of the bars to the other. On top of that, this animal had a mean keeper who occasionally whipped it. So when the animal got to the part of the cage where the keeper usually stood, it flinched, even if the keeper wasn't there. The old zookeeper told me that the mean keeper was fired and when the new zoo was built this was the first animal they put into a natural habitat. She said she will never forget the day that they used a big crane that they had to ship all the way from St. Louis to move the cage into its new environment. The workman unscrewed the bars of the cage and scampered across the moat, pulling the ladder back and all of a sudden the crane pulled the cage up. The animal looked around and walked 15 yards to the left where the bars used to be and stopped and turned around and walked 15 yards to the right to where the other bars used to be. To this day, he continues to do this, flinching each time he passes the part of the bars where the mean keeper used to stand."

What kind of animal did you imagine when you read this last story? We purposely use the word "animal" in this story so that the recipient of the story can imagine any animal that will match his or her own personal realities.

The next story can be particularly useful if a patient complains of a bodily "knot" or that he or she feels "tied up in knots." Suppose our patient is named "Jane."

"Jane, a couple of months ago, I ran into an old friend of mine named Joan. She and I were talking about many things and then Joan told me an interesting story: She remembered how years ago when she was just a little girl, she was walking around the harbor with her parents and a nice old tugboat captain gave her an interesting-looking piece of rope. He told her that rope had traveled the Seven Seas and he suggested that she take it home and have fun with it. Joan was playing with her new toy later that day and was enjoying swinging it in the air and cracking it like a whip, but then she accidentally knocked something over. One of her parents came in screaming at her and they tied her rope into tight knots and threw it out the door and told her to get out there where she belonged. Joan was walking around sadly outside with her new toy all tied up in knots and then she sat down next to a nice old neighbor lady who had done a lot of sailing. As Joan watched closely, the neighbor was able to *untie the first knot, Jane,* and then the neighbor gave the rope back to Joan. The neighbor told Joan to play with the rope outside with that first knot untied and to learn more about the rope and then, remembering what she had seen, she would be able to *untie the next knot.* Joan was told to play with the rope some more, and to learn just how to have fun with it safely and then she would be able to *untie the next knot, Jane.* Then the neighbor told Joan to take the rope back inside, and to be careful at first and to learn just when and where she could play with the rope in there and then she would be able to *untie the next knot.* Joan was told that soon she would have all the knots in that rope untied, and would be playing with that rope lots of times, in lots of places, and would be able to *have a lot of fun, Jane.* Then, before Joan left, the nice neighbor leaned over and whispered an important secret into Joan's ear. Joan left, and after playing with the rope for a while, and remembering just what she had seen and heard, she was able to *untie the next knot.* She played with the rope some more and then she was able to *untie the next knot.* She went back inside with the rope, and carefully started to learn just when and where she could play with the rope, and then she was able to *untie the next knot.* Soon she had all the knots in that rope untied, and was playing with the rope a lot and she told me that she was able to *have a lot of fun, Jane.* When my friend told me that story about the knot, I was rather curious and asked her what that secret was that the nice old neighbor told her. Well, Joan just looked at me and smiled, and said, 'Charlie, it's a secret. I can't tell you what it is, but I'll bet that in some kind of way you know.' Well, maybe I do, and maybe you do too."

This story communicated a suggestion to Jane to untie the knots within herself. Note that the friend's name in the story has the same first letter as the patient's name, and note also that the embedded suggestions in the story—"untie the first knot, Jane," "have a lot of fun, Jane," and so on—substitute Jane's name for the person in the story. This makes no logical sense, but it is surprising how patients will never notice this grammatical error when embedded suggestions are communicated like this. The above therapeutic story also utilizes the strategy of accessing the patient's own unconscious resources for problem resolution (when the neighbor tells Jane a *secret*).

Constructing a Metaphorical Story

Many of the people who have written about therapeutic metaphors (for example, Lankton & Lankton, 1983) have turned a relatively easy and enjoyable technique into a difficult task by suggesting many technical requirements for such construction. Some of the simplest stories, like the two-dog story, get the best results. We have three suggestions to help you learn to construct stories. First, and probably most important, remember that the power of therapeutic storytelling is increased by utilizing within the story symbols or metaphors that belong to the patient. Listen closely during intake to how each patient expresses himself or herself. Notice what is happening in his or her life, including interests and hobbies. Do not tell a man who likes baseball but has no interest in gardens a story about flower gardens, for it will not pique his interest. If a patient is bothered by dermatological problems or allergies (even if that is not the presenting problem) make up a story about something or someone who gets under another's skin and how it can be dealt with. If your patient suffers from headaches, then include someone or something in your story that's "a big headache" for the story's hero. Or if a patient has gastrointestinal (GI) problems, talk about how the hero has had difficulty "swallowing," "stomaching," or "digesting" what is going on. It is likely that a patient with GI symptoms would use such metaphors. Be creative in your storytelling so as not to be too obvious that you are really talking about the patient.

Second, the therapist can use his or own images of patients to construct stories. After the patient leaves your office for the first time, close your eyes and see what images appear. These images can provide interesting guidance. If the patient appears to be a wimpering puppy, go with it in your story. Third, have fun and do not worry that the patient may see through the story you develop. If he or she does, you lose the value of indirect communication, but the patient might still see your story as an interesting parallel example concerning his or her problem: no harm is done to the therapy process.

An Existential View of the Addiction Problem

We wanted this text to include a detailed discussion of one diagnostic entity to give the reader a sense of some of the ways an existentially oriented professional would view a particular diagnostic label and related patient behaviors. For reasons we will discuss at the end of the next paragraph, we chose the "addiction" label to address in some detail. The general issues, however, are applicable to most of the behaviors and labels any hypnotherapist deals with.

THEORY

In the 1970s and most of the '80s Americans viewed the disease of addiction and its treatment in a mostly one-dimensional way: treat the alcohol or drug abuser by means of a 28-day detox inpatient stay, and follow up hospitalization with drug and alcohol outpatient counseling and one of the many so-called 12-step programs. The practice of hypnotherapy was rarely involved as part of the treatment. Two recent trends changed that. First, the concept of "addictive behavior" gradually broadened to include all manner of self-abusive activities involving food, cigarettes, relationships, sex, and even jogging. Second, the extremely high per-patient cost, coupled with only modest success, of inpatient treatment has stimulated the insurance industry to begin requiring alternative forms of treatment, the most common of which is outpatient psychotherapy with a licensed practitioner. Many of these clinicians use hypnosis as part of their treatment because some of their clients view it as an attractive alternative to "talking psychotherapy." Therefore we have included a special chapter on this one clinical entity partly because it is such a new and rapidly growing segment of the patient population for hypnotherapists, but also because the new, broader concept of "addiction" poses some particularly interesting theoretical and clinical problems from the perspective of an existentially oriented clinician.

Some time ago we were conducting a training workshop for professionals who worked with adult children of alcoholics. At the end of the workshop we were criticized by two of the female participants who said that we were professionally negligent for making food available during the workshop breaks. These two women experienced themselves as "food addicts" and were in the Overeaters Anonymous program, which requires total abstinence from food between meals. They complained that as professionals in the addiction field we should have known better, and they told us that because we made food available, our action forced them during the breaks of our workshop to go into the bathroom and recite the "Serenity Prayer" a dozen times in order to gain enough strength not to eat. Many months after this incident we were still bothered, not by the specific complaints of these women, but by our own unwillingness to take them seriously. We had always viewed ourselves as compassionate human beings who were willing to listen seriously to anyone in pain; yet we had no sympathy for these women. Finally, while discussing this incident, we realized that the reason we did not take these women seriously was that they never asked us to take them seriously. Rather, they demanded that we take their self-imposed label as "food addicts" seriously.

Labeling and self-labeling is the first problem of the commonly accepted addiction model. For too many people the label tends to become the whole definition of the self: I am an alcoholic, I am an adult child of an alcoholic, I am an addict. This is particularly true with people who participate in a 12-step recovery program because generally each time they speak at a meeting they introduce themselves by saying "Hi, I am Mark and I am an alcoholic," or "Hi, I am Joan and I am an addict." Mark may well be an alcoholic, but he might also be a college professor, a husband, a father, a terrific fly fisherman, and so on, and Jane might well be an addict, but also an excellent nurse, a wife, a devoted mother, and a champion bowler. Unfortunately, the "I am the addict" or "I am the alcoholic" label gets repeated, day in and day out, meeting after meeting, and becomes for that person the most important definition of himself or herself. This is a problem because such a definition is not only narrow and limiting, but also pathological.

Second, labels make people into objects. An object is always what it is labeled: it can never change. A pencil is always a pencil. It may be a sharp pencil or a dull pencil, with or without an eraser, in use or lying still, but it is always a pencil. Yet being human means being different in different circumstances. People are coconstituted by their world.[1] We are teachers only during these times that we interact with people willing to be students. At other times we are students helping to coconstitute the teacher in that situation who in fact is coconstituting us as students. When people constantly give themselves the same label over and over again, they are reducing themselves to a thinglike existence, and in this case a particularly pathological existence.

The third problem with the notion of labels is that all labels can only be understood as general categories at best. There are many different kinds of cancer, such that any two people with "cancer" can be radically different in terms of the symptoms and prognosis of their disease. Likewise, any two children raised in homes with an alcoholic parent will have radically different experiences. In one home the alcoholic parent may be very abusive and unpredictably destructive, while in the other home the alcoholic parent may reduce the optimum functioning of the family only in a minor way. To label all children who grow up with an alcoholic parent as "children of alcoholics" and to think that they share so many

---

[1]See Chapter 1 for more detailed discussion of coconstitutionality.

characteristics that these shared characteristics overwhelm individual differences misses the point. Often an adult child of an alcoholic will be more similar in upbringing and personality characteristics to a person raised in a home without alcohol than he or she is to another adult child of an alcoholic. Too many clinicians miss that reality because of their "addiction" to labels and the illusion of understanding people by grouping them into broad categories of being.

It is very seductive, yet dangerous, to make complex phenomena simple by giving them labels that we think we understand. In politics we often elect very bad leaders because we tend to label political positions as "liberal" or "conservative," and then vote for people based on the appeal of the particular label. Similarly, therapists and other health professionals often *mis*treat many patients by employing a standard treatment that they think belongs to a particular label, and therefore fail to treat the real person and his or her own individual idiosyncratic needs. Indeed, labels cause us to misunderstand people every bit as much as they help us to understand what goes on. As Sigmund Freud (1963, p. 87) said, "We know that the first step toward intellectual mastery of the world is the discovery of general principles, rules and laws which bring order into chaos. By such mental operations we simplify the world, but we could not avoid falsifying it in doing so, especially because we are dealing with processes of development and change." Or as Hermann Hesse (1974, p. 94), the existential novelist, writes, "Clarity and truth are often used side-by-side as if they more or less belong together. Rarely is truth clear and even more rarely is clarity true. The truth is always complex, obscure, and ambiguous—every clear statement does violence towards the truth."

Another problem with the use of labels is that for someone with an existential orientation *being* always implies *being-toward-a future*. Once we label someone—whether ourselves or others—those labels seem resistant to change. Carl Rogers (1947) demonstrated this truth with his research on self-concept. He showed that once one's self-concept is formed it becomes resistant to change even if change results in improvement. Rosenhan (1973) in his classic study also found the same thing in regard to diagnostic labels. This is particularly a problem in the addiction field because the basic model used in the 12-step process includes the belief "once an addict, always an addict." Today recovering alcoholics in the Alcoholics Anonymous program believe that 15 years from now, even if they have not taken a single drink in the interim, they will still be alcoholics and will still be in serious jeopardy even if they take a single drink. Think of the lack of personal power that is implied by the notion that 15 years from now one drink can still get you. It seems to us that the ultimate recovery program is one that leads to the discovery of empowerment: this is where the 12-step model falls short. In fact, it is our belief that the 12-step model is really no more than a first step in that positive movement toward the future of personal power and enrichment. We believe people need to be free *for* something rather than free *from* something. A true existential addiction model requires understanding the alcoholic or other addiction process differently so that the label has a requirement of change associated with it. The end goal of existential therapy, personal power and free choice, would then be in sight at all times.

Sociologists such as Lemert (1951), Goffman (1961), and Becker (1963) have long recognized the dire consequences of the labeling process. They describe, for example, how a person might identify with a deviant label (for example, "drug addict" or "junkie") and then use drugs in an increased way to deal with feelings of poor self-esteem, guilt, and anxiety augmented by the application of that label. The situation is made worse by society's aversive reaction to the negative label, which only increases the addict's poor self-esteem and anxiety, and which may, in fact, support the addict's need to use drugs to cope and to believe that he or she only fits in with other addicts. Likewise, "criminals" often find it very difficult to put their criminal pasts behind them because the stigma of their label prevents them from getting decent legitimate jobs and drives them deeper into criminal careers in order to survive. Certainly, the application of deviant labels will often decrease a person's ability to find opportunities for being responsible and therefore strengthen his or her feelings of personal power.

Another major problem with the addiction model is that the widespread use of this model takes people "off the hook" for some of their behavior and does it in a way that reduces them to children. In Chapter 1 we quoted Willie Nelson's song "Black Rose": "The devil made me do it the first time, the second time I done it on my own." From an existential perspective this model is much healthier than the current addiction model that says "The first time I did it on my own (though I was influenced by peers, advertising, and so on), but thereafter I was addicted and couldn't help myself." Owning a self-destructive behavior has to be a better way to make changes than the powerlessness associated with the first step of the Alcoholics Anonymous program.[2] This change in position may help many patients to bypass a 28-day hospitalization and a lifetime of meetings. Let us say something loud and clear: We understand that some people will not or cannot take the decision to assert personal power. It is clearly better for such people to admit their powerlessness over the substance they abuse and to get help in the way that it is traditionally given than it is for them to continue the abuse of the substance and the social disruption that goes with it. We admit that the addiction treatment model that is currently used is very helpful for many people and may be the only treatment mode that some people can use. But we also believe (1) that there are alternative models that might work better for *some* people; and (2) that the traditional addiction model, however good it is, does have side effects, especially the encouragement of powerlessness, that need to be considered.

Clearly, many people use the "addiction" label for permission to abdicate personal responsibility. As we noted in Chapter 1, one of the major goals of existential psychotherapy is to bring the patient to a psychological position of per-

---

[2]The first step of Alcoholics Anonymous (1976, p. 59) states, "We admitted we were powerless over alcohol—that our lives had become unmanageable."

sonal responsibility. Simply put, therapy ends when patients see themselves as voluntary participants in, rather than as victims of, the situation and are willing to mobilize their personal power to change their lives.

The crutch of lack of personal responsibility for one's behavior is very clearly demonstrated in the widespread belief that cigarette smoking is maintained by an "addiction" to nicotine. This notion is promoted by health professionals even though much of the literature in the field demonstrates a positive correlation between the belief a person has that he or she is addicted and the difficulty he or she will have in stopping smoking (Gritz, 1980). The fact is that tens of millions of people have stopped smoking, some easily and most without professional help. A high percentage of "addicted" women smokers manage to stop the day they find out they have conceived a child and they manage to refrain from smoking throughout the pregnancy and nursing period, even if they do take up the habit again later on. No nicotine addiction theory can explain this truth. Likewise, millions of people who practice an Orthodox religion and who claim they cannot go 2 hours without a cigarette voluntarily stop smoking on holy days. Such things as smoking and nonsmoking behaviors can all be better understood in light of existential concepts of meaning and choice than by a substance abuse explanation. A detailed critique of the addiction–cigarette link is well beyond the scope of this book; however, one example should help to clarify the problem. The introduction to *Smoking and Health: A Report of the Surgeon General* (U.S. Department of Health, Education and Welfare, 1976) officially declares cigarette smoking is addictive. The Surgeon General highlights three factors from the literature that in his mind clearly demonstrate the validity of this conclusion. One of these factors is a group of surveys that ask people if they would like to stop smoking. Each survey reports an affirmative answer ranging from 95 to 99%. The Surgeon General then concludes that if all these smokers would like to stop and do not, they must be addicted. The problem with this conclusion is that in the actual literature none of the surveys asked the respondent, "Do you want to stop smoking?" What the surveys asked was,

"Would you like to stop smoking if it were easy?" We have always wondered what the responses would be if the question asked, "Would you like to stop even if it were very difficult but you could?" Our guess is that a lot fewer people would answer "Yes." In working with patients it is always important to find out what they mean by words like "want" and "try." Does it mean they *want* to do something very badly and will *try* even when it is difficult or are those just words that are easily thrown around? Last night we watched television. We wanted to read Plato and Socrates, but we were tired so we watched television. Are we addicted to television just because we "wanted" to do something else, yet watched the tube instead? The surveys mentioned above tell us a lot about the American public, but not much about addiction or nicotine.

In *Siddhartha* Hermann Hesse (1951) writes that you can do whatever you want to do if you are willing to "think, wait, and fast." The first two of these notions are self-evident. Thinking, using your mind, and waiting, having some patience, obviously are important requirements for personal success. What we believe he means by the third directive, "fast," is to have discipline and be willing to work to do what is difficult. Clients too must be taught to understand that achieving success means in developing a willingness to own the possibility of success and working hard to achieve it. If just wanting success were enough, everyone would be a winner. Many times the patients we know are engaging in behavior that is either stupid or lazy and they need to own up to that truth so they can make changes. Allowing them to think that their behavior is caused by an addiction as opposed to their own will is counterproductive to encouraging growth and change. In a paradoxical way, the addiction model often does what it claims drugs do; that is, it takes freedom away from people.

A recent widespread, and we think bizarre, element relative to the addiction model has been the inclusion of behavior such as sexuality, eating, and even jogging in this category. All manner of activities are now lumped together into the catch-all category of "behavioral drugs." The simple fact is that if you have been told by your doctor to stop jogging because it is bad for your knees; you have made a few attempts to do so, but in fact keep jogging because it feels good or because your friends do it; then this behavior would basically fit into the DSM-III-R (American Psychiatric Association, 1987) criteria for addiction. This is a one-item test of how bizarre this classification business has become.

Two basic trends in the literature seem to explain these so-called addictions, both of which not only take away personal power from people but also dehumanize them. The first of these trends is a framework that states that personally or interpersonally destructive behaviors basically stem from low self-concept originating in poor early childhood experiences (the most popular of these being the codependence and adult child of alcoholics syndromes). The second trend says that such behaviors are maintained by physiological responses such as norepenephrine or endorphin release during these activities. This belief reduces people to bundles of dysfunctional physiological responses. We have worked in our own private practices with many cigarette smokers and we have never met anyone who sits down for a "hit of nicotine." Most of the time people just want to smoke a cigarette. It is true that *some*times *some* people will get up in the morning with the intention to alert themselves with the nicotine intake of a cigarette: this is the personal meaning that this cigarette has for them. However, a few hours later, stressed out at work, they may want to relax and will have a "relaxing" cigarette. Now the smoker will almost never think of nicotine because the notion of taking in speed (nicotine) to relax is opposed to the belief most people have about nicotine. Reducing complex human behaviors such as smoking, human sexuality, eating, or whatever, to simple physiological cravings and responses is opposed to the most basic beliefs of existential philosophy and psychology, especially as far as the concepts of personal choice and responsibility are concerned.

A major problem with using the addiction model to treat all these other problem behaviors is that we now have groups of people who are basically untrained in psychodynamics and in treating patients for complex personal and interpersonal problems who are in fact doing such treatment. Just because someone is a certified addiction counselor and has some experience using a 12-step model to treat drug and alcohol addiction does not mean that that person is qualified to do marriage counseling with couples in which one partner is having affairs just because "having affairs" has been labeled an addictive sexual behavior.

Everyone working in the addiction field knows the "Serenity Prayer" written by Reinhold Niebuhr:

> God grant me the serenity to accept the things I cannot change,
> Courage to change the things I can,
> And the wisdom to know the difference.

This prayer begins or ends almost every 12-step meeting and clearly offers some helpful wisdom, at least in theory. In practice, however, what we have noticed is that most people focus on the first line and give themselves permission to accept many things that perhaps they do not need to accept. One example is the women we discussed at the beginning of this chapter who, rather than just saying no to the food at our workshops and feeling good about it, instead had to run to the bathroom and repeatedly recite this prayer. What we believe has happened for many people is that the concept of addiction itself has blocked the "wisdom to know the difference." As we tried to make clear in Chapter 1, what you believe to be true will become your truth. If you believe you are "addicted" then you usually will also believe that it will be very difficult to stop or change that behavior and therefore the difficulty will likely exist for you. As we noted earlier, people who believe that they are addicted to nicotine will be less likely to try to stop smoking; if they do try to stop, they will have more severe withdrawal symptoms (Gritz, 1980). In fact, for most substance withdrawal the best predictor of the severity of the symptoms of that withdrawal will be the belief the person has about what the withdrawal symptoms are likely to be. We would like to rewrite the "Serenity Prayer" as follows:

God grant me the serenity to accept the things I cannot change,
COURAGE TO CHANGE THE THINGS I CAN,
And the wisdom to know the difference.

It is our hope that the theory and techniques discussed in this text will encourage a psychotherapy that gives people an understanding that they *can* change most things in their life, even to some degree other people's behavior as it affects them by changing their response to that behavior.

We know that classification of pathology in general has some value. It does give professionals a handle on some of the complex phenomena in front of them and a roadmap about the best way treatment can proceed. It can be a communication tool between professionals that can also be helpful. The notion of addiction as a classification has value. As we have previously stated, millions of lives have been saved by the current addiction model and subsequent related treatment including 12-step programs such as Alcoholics Anonymous. Though in theory it is not necessarily so, in practice we see that the *side effect of a powerlessness ideology* (not over a substance but over one's life) is a high percentage of people who believe themselves to be addicted even after their pathological behavior has stopped. As this book argues, we believe this outcome is no small sacrifice; therefore, we urge use of an addiction model only when it is absolutely necessary in the same way that you would give chemotherapy to a patient only when you are sure that they have a kind of cancer that would require such a treatment because of the severe side effects.

The so-called big book by Dr. Bob and Bill W. (Alcoholics Anonymous, 1976) was written in 1939. There is almost no subject that we do not know more about today in the 1990s than we did in 1939. However, many people still treat the first AA book as if it was the Bible and not subject to revision. Maybe the 12-step program needs a 13th or a 14th step or maybe it can be done better with 8 steps, 3 of which are different than the steps now being used. Maybe it does not matter what the steps are. The brilliant idea that made AA so successful might be just that it offered numbered steps to success. Many people in our culture love to have order and the numbering system gives many a sense of knowing where they are and where they are going in treatment. While respecting the anonymity of the participants (as in any research population), we need to do more research about 12-step programs. Yet the people in these programs seem to be hostile to the idea of examination. A very high percentage of workers in this field are recovering themselves, and such people seem to need to believe that *their* way of recovery is the *only* way. Therefore, they are not open in an honest, intellectual, and scientifically valid way to investigating alternatives. We are well aware of the very prevalent notion in the field of alcoholism and drug abuse of the loss-of-control phenomenon and the associated disease concept of addiction. Such frameworks emphasize physical variables such as genetic tendencies, long-term blood chemistry, and brain structure and/or functioning changes. These frameworks seem always to conclude that it is nearly impossible for a once-addicted person to be engaged in controlled use of his or her abused substance. Many theories say controlled use of any substance with abuse potential is impossible. We suggest that professionals with this viewpoint open their eyes. Tens of thousands of people are functioning very well today who were once diagnosed as addicted and who are now engaged in controlled use of a substance. Some addiction experts argue this point by explaining the controlled-use phrase as "preaddiction." This is like saying that skiing is a pre-broken-leg behavior. Existentialists have no trouble understanding this issue. If over time the meaning of the drug-taking behavior changes for a person, that person is engaging in a different behavior. The behavior that at one time disrupted the person's life and seemed out of control may at a later time be an unimportant event or even a healthy behavior.

We wish to restate our theme: most of the existential issues discussed in regard to addictive behaviors are applicable to all clinical diagnostic categories and to the very idea of labeling itself. Here we have detailed one classification group, the so-called addictions, only to facilitate a more detailed discussion of the issues. Clearly, the professional's use of labels and categorization to promote his or her illusion of understanding the patient and an existential psychology do not easily coexist.

TREATMENT

In existential hypnotherapy the treatment for an addiction problem should utilize all the understandings and techniques discussed elsewhere in this text. The desired outcome for all patients is a sense of empowerment and responsibility. With this outcome some patients will be able to use a previously harmful substance in a controlled way, but some will need to choose never again to use the substance. It is probably safer for a patient to decide never again to use a substance, but it is up to each patient to discover what his or her own needs are and what he or she needs to do to meet these needs.

Chapter 6, on the personal meaning of symptoms, is partially relevant to these disorders. Patients need to discover healthy alternative ways to meet their needs. All the hypnotic techniques of empowerment, including anchoring and visualization, as well as the anxiety management techniques discussed in Chapter 5, are important. We try not to use the concept of "addiction" with our patients. A concept is not a thing unto itself: it is only a way of understanding a phenomenon. For many people in our culture the addiction concept comes with some particularly heavy baggage. For example, most people believe that all addictions have associated severe withdrawal symptoms. Since expectation is always a significant factor for any outcome, we give patients the message that change will be easier than they expect. We also give patients the hypnotic message that *when* they change their behavior, *then* they will experience a sense of personal power that will make the change easier and more useful to them than they thought possible. Sometimes in treatment we actually challenge a patient's use of the word "addiction," especially when we perceive that the patient is using this label as a means of abdicating personal responsibility for uncontrolled, unhealthy behavior. For example, here is some communication rendered during hypnotic trance to one woman cigarette smoker who talked at the start of treatment about her "addiction" to cigarettes and how difficult that had made it for her to stop smoking:

"Jan, earlier, you said you had an addiction to cigarettes and that's why it had been so tough for you to stop smoking. I wasn't exactly sure what you meant by that because I know that it can be quite confusing just what an addiction is. You said it was very difficult for you to stop smoking because every time you did, you felt very irritable, but I know that any time just about anyone stops doing something that they're real used to doing they feel irritated. For example, a friend of mine used to jog every day at five o'clock but one week he wasn't able to jog. He told me that he felt so irritated around five o'clock that week that he figured that he had to be addicted to jogging. I've seen all kinds of complex things happen with these so-called addictions, even with heroin. I remember years ago, when I was working with heroin users, it was quite common that if one of our patients thought his or her methadone during detox was reduced too much that patient would go into physical withdrawal, even when the methadone hadn't been lowered at all. It was obvious that there was a psychological aspect to all this, so we decided at that program just not to tell the patient when his or her methadone was being reduced and that seemed to help him or her not to have withdrawal as seriously. I remember one time when someone who was in prison was being released after 20 years and even though he may have used a little contraband heroin behind bars now and then, there was no way he could be physically addicted to heroin. But when he went back to his old street corner where he used to buy and use a lot of drugs, he went into physical withdrawal. We took him to the emergency room and the doctor there said he was showing all the signs and symptoms of withdrawal from heroin, even though he hadn't used any and all he had done was go back to that street corner. These kinds of happenings are well known among heroin users and clinicians who treat them. Now I know that things can also be complex when it comes to cigarettes or nicotine. For example, even though some people have difficulty giving up cigarettes, most of us know people who have stopped smoking rather easily, even though they were smoking two or three packs a day. I know that I have asked a lot of women like yourself, Jan, if they thought it would be difficult to stop smoking if the lives of their children depended on their stopping and just about every one of them stated it would be no problem at all to stop under those circumstances. And since you talk so lovingly about your children, I bet that you would say the same thing, Jan. So, it seems like there's a strong psychological aspect to cigarette smoking and that may be why something like hypnosis is so helpful, Jan."

Instead of using the word "addiction," we use phrases such as "unhealthy habit" or "dysfunctional habit," or "unhealthy pattern of behavior." However, if a patient uses the term "addiction" and seems firmly commited to this usage, we will not fight or argue about it. A hallmark of effective communication or of hypnosis is to not fight or argue with a patient but to utilize the patient's realities to help lead the person to a healthier place. In fact, we will even support, on occasion, an "addicted" smoker's use of nicotine-replacement chewing gum or a nicotine patch, or an "addicted" alcoholic's use of Antabuse as a part of treatment. Again, we rely on strategies like these only when the patient strongly believes that they will be helpful. Of course, we would also do Tibetan chants during trance if our patient strongly believed that would be helpful.

For a more detailed discussion of a hypnotic approach to the treatment of smoking and overeating (and in a limited way alcohol), we refer the reader to our earlier book, *Modern Clinical Hypnosis for Habit Control* (Citrenbaum et al., 1985).

CHAPTER 9

The Woods

We have a friend named Toni who grew up on a farm located at the edge of a beautiful redwood forest. Toni told us one day about how when she was a child she discovered a path in the woods that led to a beautiful meadow overlooking the lake and how when she became 4 or 5 years old she took that path every day. At first she went down the path to the meadow with her imaginary friend, and later she took her real friends with her. When she grew older she took her dates there. She even told us about her first sexual experiences in that meadow overlooking that lake. Later, as a young adult, she went sometimes with a friend to talk, sometimes just with a book to read, or even without a book to meditate. She talked not only of the meadow and the lake but of the path, all the flowers, the friendly animals along the way that she visited.

As Toni grew older so did the woods. The path became partially blocked by trees and branches that were knocked down during windstorms. Unfamiliar animals appeared and from time to time scared her. Toni told us that it became more and more difficult to go down that path because she would stumble now and then over a dip in the path or trip over a fallen tree. One day she walked down it carelessly and fell over. A rock had somehow gotten on the path and when she got up a rodent ran over her foot. As she jumped back she scratched herself on a thorny bush. That day, for the first time in many years, she ran out of the woods and never did make it to her meadow. The next day she came to the start of her path and was filled with mixed feelings, fear of the rodents

157

and thorns and holes in the path and yet desiring to go to her place. As she stood frozen and undecided she told us that an incredible thing happened: a mean, ugly ogre jumped out of the bushes and said, "Let me get on your back. I'll scare away all the rodents. I'll push away all the thorny bushes." Toni did not know what to do. She thought it would be unpleasant to have this ogre on her back and yet she wanted to go down the path and was afraid to do so on her own. So she said "Yes" to the ogre and he jumped on her back and kept his promise. He kept away all the rodents, but he also scared away all the friendly animals. He knocked aside all the thorny bushes, but he also pushed away the soft ones she liked to touch. Even though Toni was able to get to her favorite spot she felt weighed down; the journey was not enjoyable like it used to be.

For many days whenever Toni came to the start of her path the ogre jumped out and said, "Let me get on your back." Because she could not think of an alternative, she always said, "Yes." Although carrying the ogre became more and more unpleasant for her, she continued to do it because she wanted to go to her spot. One day she asked a neighbor what to do about this problem and the neighbor said, "I can't help you but nobody knows more about the woods than the Jaguar Lady who is camped down around the other side of the woods and over two small mountains and across three valleys." One day Toni packed a lunch and for the first time instead of going down her path walked around the edge of the woods and over the two mountains and across the three valleys until she came to an old lady hunched over a fire chanting a strange song.

After a while the Jaguar Lady noticed Toni and said, "Yes, my child?" And then Toni proceeded to tell her the story about her path in the woods and her favorite place and all that she had been able to do there. She also told her how the path had become overgrown and told her about the thorns and logs and rodents, and then she told her the incredible story about the ogre. The Jaguar Lady listened patiently and when Toni had finished the whole story the Jaguar Lady said:

"Sit down. I have some things to tell you, my child. The woods have many paths. There are others that would probably lead to your meadow and others that lead to different places and in their own way are just as good and maybe better. I know the woods can be scary and I imagine that you can feel fear and anxiety at the thought of taking an unknown path, yet facing that fear and moving toward the unknown is where your spiritual growth lies. In a way the overgrown path and knocked-down logs, the thorny bushes and, yes, even the rodents, are the wood's gifts to you. Without them such a gift would be too easy. To continue on a safe and comfortable path you would only experience your one spot in the woods throughout your life. You could pass through this life and only have a very limited view of your beloved woods. When you go home, move forward, face your own anxiety, and experience different paths. Some will be rewarding to you and some will not, but there will be many pleasant surprises and much personal growth along the way."

Then Toni said, "What about the ogre?" The Jaguar Lady continued:

"My child, there have been many times in your life when you have attempted to do things and things came out just the way you wanted them to or even surprisingly better. When you were able to feel confident, competent, powerful, on top of the world like there was nothing you couldn't do. Remember one of those times right now and as you remember it take the thumb and your middle finger of your right hand and squeeze them together so that you can feel the power of those fingers meeting as you remember that moment of personal power in your history. The next time you go into the woods and you see your ogre, look him in the eye, put your thumb and middle finger together, remember that moment of power, and tell the ogre, 'No!' Tell him to get off your back. You'll have to say it like you mean it and you'll have to say it a few times, but once the ogre knows you mean it the ogre will leave: they always do."

When the Jaguar Lady finished talking she put her head down and began chanting the strange song again. Toni got up, mumbled a thank you, and went back across the three valleys and over the two mountains to her home. The next day she went out to the woods and saw another path that she had passed many times before but had never taken and decided today she would take this one, even though she felt nervous in even saying that to herself. Just as she came to the foot of the path the ogre jumped out and said, "Let me get on your back. I'll scare away the rodents and knock away the thorns on this path for you too." Toni remembered what the Jaguar Lady had said. She pushed her thumb and middle finger together and that seemed to remind her of her own history of power and she looked at the ogre and said, "No!" The ogre said, "Come on, let me get on your back. I can help you again!" Toni just looked him right in the eye and said, "No! No! No!" Then the ogre left. Toni tried that path but did not enjoy it very much. There was no clearing for her to sit down in on that path and there were not many beautiful flowers or soft bushes. The next day she saw another path that appeared to be really scary because it seemed to go down a deep hill. Just as she stood at the foot of that path, feeling very nervous about this potential new experience, the ogre jumped out and once again said, "Today, let me get on your back. I'll help you down this hill." Toni just looked him in the eye and put her thumb and middle finger together and with as much conviction as she had ever had said, "Not on your life, never again!" The ogre left and Toni never saw him again. It turned out that there are three or four paths she takes now. Every once in a while she finds a different one that she has never ever taken before and tries it.

And that is the story of our friend Toni and the woods. Of course, this story really has nothing to do with you because after all she is our friend not yours, but then again. . . .

References

Alcoholics Anonymous. (1976, June). New York: Alcoholics Anonymous World Services.

American Psychiatric Association. (1987). *Diagnostic and Statistical Manual of Mental Disorders* (3rd ed., rev.). Washington, DC: American Psychiatric Association.

Andreas, C., & Andreas, S. (1987). *Change Your Mind and Keep the Change.* Moab, UT: Real People Press.

Bandler, R. (1985). *Using Your Brain for a Change.* Moab, UT: Real People Press.

Bandler, R., & Grinder, J. (1979). *Frogs into Princes.* Moab, UT: Real People Press.

Barber, J. (1980). Hypnosis and the unhypnotizable. *American Journal of Clinical and Experimental Hypnosis, 23,* 4–9.

Barker, P. (1985). *Using Metaphors in Psychotherapy.* New York: Brunner/Mazel.

Bateson, M. C. (1991, November). *Composing a Life.* Paper presented at the 11th Annual Common Boundary Conference on Sacred Stories, Arlington, VA.

Becker, H. S. (1963). *Outsiders.* New York: The Free Press.

Bennett, D. (1989, May). *Human Consciousness as a Virtual Von Neumann Machine.* Paper presented at the conference on Philosophy, Neurology and Artificial Intelligence, School of Medicine, University of Pittsburgh.

Berne, E. (1961). *Transactional Analysis in Psychotherapy.* New York: Grove Press.

Bettelheim, B. (1977). *The Uses of Enchantment.* New York: Vintage Books.

Booth, L., Fr. (1992, July). *Saying Yes to Life: Spirituality—You Can't Recover without It.* Keynote address, 11th Avenue Florida School of Addiction Studies, Tampa, FL.

Bradshaw, J. (1990). *Homecoming.* New York: Bantam.

Braid, J. (1843). *Neurypnology: Or the Rationale of Nervous Sleep Considered in Relation with Animal Magnetism.* London. (Referenced in Pettinati, H. (Ed.). (1980). *Hypnosis and Memory* (Chapter 5). New York: Guilford Press.)

Capacchione, L. (1991). *Recovery of Your Inner Child.* New York: Simon & Schuster.

Carpenter, A. E. (1900). *Plain Instructions in Hypnotism and Mesmerism.* Boston: Lee & Shepard/Rockwell & Churchill Press.

Citrenbaum, C. M., King, M. E., & Cohen, W. I. (1985). *Modern Clinical Hypnosis for Habit Control.* New York: W. W. Norton.

Diamond, M. J. (1984). It takes two to tango: Some thoughts on the neglected importance of the hypnotist in an interactive hypnotherapeutic relationship. *American Journal of Clinical and Experimental Hypnosis, 27,* 3–13.

Diamond, M. J. (1987). The interactional basis of hypnotic experience: In the relational dimensions of hypnosis. *International Journal of Clinical and Experimental Hypnosis, 35,* 95–115.

Diamond, S., & Beaumont, J. (1974). *Hemisphere Function in the Human Brain.* New York: Halstead Press/John Wiley & Sons.

Erickson, M. H. (1966). The interspersal hypnotic technique for symptom correction and pain control." *American Journal of Clinical Hypnosis, 3,* 198–209.

Erickson, M. H. (1980). *The Collected Papers of Milton H. Erickson* (4 vols.) (E. L. Rossi, Ed.). New York: Irvington.

Erickson, M. H. (1983). *Healing in Hypnosis* (E. L. Rossi, M. O. Ryan, & F. L. Sharp, Eds.). New York: Irvington.

Erickson, M. H., & Rossi, E. (Eds.). (1976a). *Hypnotic Realities.* New York: Irvington.

Erickson, M. H., & Rossi, E. (1976b). Two-level communications and the microdynamics of trance. *American Journal of Clinical Hypnosis, 18,* 153–171.

Erickson, M. H., & Rossi, E. (1979). *Hypnotherapy: An Exploratory Casebook.* New York: Irvington.

Erikson, E. H. (1968). *Identity: Youth and Crisis.* New York: W. W. Norton.

Fagen, J., & Shepherd, I. (1970). *Gestalt Therapy Now.* Palo Alto, CA: Science & Behavior Books.

Feinstein, D., & Krippner, S. (1988). *Personal Mythology.* New York: St. Martin's Press.

Fischer, W. (1978). *Theories of Anxiety.* New York: Harper & Row.

Fox, M. (1989, June). Original blessing, not original sin. *Psychology Today*, pp. 18–23.

Freud, S. (1949). *Outline of Psychoanalysis*. New York: W. W. Norton.

Freud, S. (1963). *Therapy and Technique*. New York: Macmillan.

Fromm, E., & Kahn, S. (1990). *Self-Hypnosis: The Chicago Paradigm*. New York: Guilford Press.

Gavitz, M. (1991). Early themes of hypnosis: A clinical perpsepctive. In S. J. Lynn & J. W. Rhue (Eds.), *Theories of Hypnosis*. New York: Guilford Press.

Goffman, E. (1961). *Asylums*. New York: Anchor Books.

Goldenson, R. M. (1984). *Longman Dictionary of Psychology and Psychiatry*. New York: Longman Press.

Gordon, D. (1978). *Therapeutic Metaphors*. Palo Alto, CA: Meta Publications.

Grinder, J., & Bandler, R. (1981). *Trance-Formations*. Moab, UT: Real People Press.

Gritz, E. (1980). *Smoking Behavior and Tobacco Abuse*. New York: JAI Press.

Grove, D. (1989). *Resolving Feelings of Anger, Guilt and Shame* (a Seminar Handbook). Edwardsville, IL: David Grove Seminars.

Haley, J. (1984). *Ordeal Therapy*. San Francisco, CA: Jossey-Bass.

Hall, J. A. (1989). *Hypnosis: A Jungian Perspective*. New York: Guilford Press.

Hammond, D. H. (1988). Will the real Milton Erickson please stand up. *International Journal of Clinical and Experimental Hypnosis*, 36, 173–181.

Harner, M. (1990). *The Way of the Shaman*. New York: Harper & Row.

Heidegger, M. (1962). *Being and Time* (J. Macquarrie & E. Robinson, Trans.). New York: Harper & Row. (Original work published 1926)

Hesse, H. (1951). *Siddhartha*. New York: New Directions.

Hesse, H. (1974). *Reflections*. New York: Farrar, Straus & Giroux.

Hilgard, E. R. (1965). *Hypnotic Susceptibility*. New York: Harcourt, Brace & World.

Hillman, J. (1975). *Re-Visioning Psychology*. New York: Harper & Row.

Hillman, J., & Ventura, M. (1992). *We've Had a Hundred Years of Theory and the World's Getting Wise*. San Francisco: Harper & Row.

Hogan, R., & Kirchner, J. (1967). Preliminary report of the extinction of learned fear in a short term implosive therapy. *Journal of Abnormal Psychology*, 72, 106–109.

Hogan, R., & Kirchner, J. (1968). Implosive, eclectic, verbal and bibliotherapy in the treatment of fears of snakes. *Behaviour Research and Therapy, 6,* 167–171.

Homer (1967). *The Odyssey* (R. Lattimore, Trans.). New York: Harper & Row.

Jung, C. G. (1964). Foreword. In D. T. Suzuki, *An Introduction to Zen Buddhism.* New York: Grove Weidenfeld.

Keen, S. (1991, November). *Your Mythic Journey: Finding Meaning in Your Life.* Paper presented at the 11th Annual Common Boundary Conference on Sacred Stories, Arlington, VA.

Keen, S., & Fox, A. V. (1973). *Telling Your Story: A Guide to Who You Are and Who You Can Be.* New York: Doubleday.

Kierkegaard, S. (1944). *The Concept of Dread* (W. Lowrie, Trans.). Princeton, NJ: Princeton University Press. (Original work published 1844)

Kierkegaard, S. (1954). *Fear and Trembling and the Sickness unto Death.* Princeton, NJ: Princeton University Press. (Original work published 1856)

King, M. E., Novik, L., & Citrenbaum, C. M. (1983). *Irresistible Communication: Creative Skills for the Health Professional.* Philadelphia: W. B. Saunders.

King, V., Golden, C. J., King, M., & Citrenbaum, C. (1989). *The Courage to Recover.* Littleton, MA: Copley Press.

Kinsbourne, M., & Smith, W. L. (Eds.). (1974). *Hemispheric Disconnection and Cerebral Function.* Springfield, IL: Charles C Thomas.

Kirmayer, L. J. (1988). Work magic and the rhetoric of common sense: Erickson's metaphors for mind. *International Journal of Clinical and Experimental Hypnosis, 36,* 157–172.

Kroger, W., & Fezler, W. (1976). *Hypnosis and Behavior Modification: Imagery Conditioning.* Philadelphia: Lippincott.

Kundera, M. (1981). *The Book of Laughter and Forgetting.* New York: Penguin Books.

Lankton, S., & Lankton C. (1983). *The Answer Within: A Clinical Framework of Ericksonian Hypnotherapy.* New York: Brunner/ Mazel.

Lazarus, A. (1984). *In the Mind's Eye.* New York: Guilford Press.

Lemert, E. (1951). *Social Pathology.* New York: McGraw-Hill.

Maslow, A. (1971). *The Farther Reaches of Human Nature.* New York: Viking Press.

Mason, A. A. (1960). *Hypnosis for Medical and Dental Practitioners.* London: Camelot Press.

May, R. (1969). *Love and Will.* New York: Dell.

May, R. (1977). *The Meaning of Anxiety*. New York: W. W. Norton.

May, R. (1981). *Freedom and Destiny*. New York: W. W. Norton.

May, R. (1989). *The Art of Counseling* (rev. ed.). New York: Gardner Press.

Miller, A. (1984). *For Your Own Good: Hidden Cruelty in Child-Rearing and the Roots of Violence*. New York: Farrar, Straus & Giroux.

Missildine, W. (1982). *Your Inner Child of the Past*. New York: Pocket Books. (Original work published 1963)

Moss, C. S., Riggen, G., Coyne, L., & Bishop, W. (1965). Some correlates of the use or disuse of hypnosis by experienced psychologists–therapists. *International Journal of Clinical and Experimental Hypnosis, 13*, 39–50.

Nietzsche, F. (1954a). Twilight of the idols. In *The Portable Nietzsche* (W. Kaufmann, Trans.). New York: Viking Press. (Original work published 1888)

Nietzsche, F. (1954b). Thus spake Zarathustra. In *The Portable Nietzsche* (W. Kaufmann, Trans). New York: Viking Press. (Original work published 1892)

Nietzsche, F. (1984). *Human, All Too Human* (M. Faber, Trans.). Lincoln, NE: University of Nebraska Press. (Original work published 1876)

Orne, M. J. (1959). The nature of hypnosis: Artifact and essence. *Journal of Abnormal and Social Psychology, 58*, 277–299.

Peck, M. S. (1978). *The Road Less Traveled*. New York: Simon & Schuster.

Perls, F. (1969). *Gestalt Therapy Verbatim*. New York: Bantam Books.

Perls, F., Hefferline, R., & Goodman, P. (1951). *Gestalt Therapy*. New York: Julian Press.

Quigley, D. (1989). *Alchemical Hypnotherapy*. Palo Alto, CA: Lost Coast Press.

Rogers, C. (1947). The organization of personality. *American Psychologist, 2*, 358–369.

Rosen, S. (1982). *My Voice Will Go with You: Teaching Tales of Milton H. Erickson*. New York: W. W. Norton.

Rosenhan, D. L. (1973). On being sane in insane places. *Science, 179*, 250–258.

Rumelhard, D. (1989, May). *Parallel Distributed Processing in Cognitive Science*. Paper presented at the conference on Philosophy, Neurology and Artificial Intelligence, School of Medicine, University of Pittsburgh.

Sartre, J.-P. (1962). *Nausea* (L. Alexander, Trans.). London: Oxford University Press. (Original work published 1938)

Sartre, J.-P. (1966). *Being and Nothingness* (H. Barnes, Trans.). London: Oxford University Press. (Original work published 1956)

Scheflin, A., & Shapiro, J. (1989). *Trance on Trial*. New York: Guilford Press.

Seltzer, L. F. (1986). *Paradoxical Strategies in Psychotherapy: A Comprehensive Overview and Guidebook*. New York: John Wiley & Sons.

Shah, I. (1971). *The Pleasantries of the Incredible Mulla Nasrudin*. New York: E. P. Dutton.

Shah, I. (1972). *The Exploits of the Incomparable Mulla Nasrudin*. New York: E. P. Dutton.

Shah, I. (1973). *The Subtleties of the Inimitable Mulla Nasrudin*. New York: E. P. Dutton.

Shor, R. E. (1959). Hypnosis and the concept of the generalized reality orientation. *American Journal of Psychotherapy, 13,* 582–602.

Shor, R. E., & Orne, M. (1962). *The Harvard Group Scale of Hypnotic Susceptibility, Form A*. Palo Alto, CA: Consulting Psychologists Press.

Simkin, J. (1976). *Gestalt Therapy Mini-Lectures*. Millbrae, CA: Celestial Arts.

Smith, M., Chu, J., & Edmonston, W. (1977). Cerebral lateralization of haptic perception. *Science, 197,* 689–690.

Spanos, N. (1991). A sociocognitive approach to hypnosis. In S. J. Lynn & J. W. Rhue (Eds.), *Theories of Hypnosis*. New York: Guilford Press.

Spiegel, H. (1974). *Manual for Hypnotic Induction Profile: Eye Roll Levitation Method*. New York: Soni Media.

Springer, S., & Deutsch, G. (1981). *Left Brain, Right Brain*. New York: W. H. Freeman.

Stampfl, T., & Levis, D. (1967). Essentials of implosive therapy: A learning theory based on psychodynamic behavioral therapy. *Journal of Abnormal Psychology, 72,* 499–503.

Suzuki, S. (1970). *Zen Mind, Beginner's Mind*. New York: Weatherhill Press.

Talmon, M. (1990). *Single Session Therapy*. San Francisco: Jossey Bass.

U.S. Department of Health, Education and Welfare. (1976). *Smoking and Health: A Report of the Surgeon General*. Washington, DC: U.S. Department of Health, Education and Welfare.

Van Dusen, W. (1960). Existential analytic psychotherapy. *American Journal of Psychoanalysis, 20,* 310–322.

Wallis, L. (1985). *Stories for the Third Ear*. New York: W. W. Norton.

Warnock, M. (1970). *Existentialism*. London: Oxford University Press.

Watzlawick, P. (1984). *The Invented Reality*. New York: W. W. Norton.

Watzlawick, P. (1985). Hypnotherapy without trance. In J. K. Zeig (Ed.), *Ericksonian Psychotherapy* (Vol. 1). New York: Brunner/Mazel.

Weitzenhoffer, A. M., & Hilgard, E. R. (1959). *Stanford Hypnotic Susceptibility Scales, Forms A and B*. Palo Alto, CA: Consulting Psychologists Press.

Whitfield, C. (1987). *Healing the Child Within*. Deerfield Beach, FL: Health Communications.

Wright, M. E., & Wright, B. A. (1987). *Clinical Practice of Hynotherapy*. New York: Guilford Press.

Yapko, M. D. (1990). *Trancework: An Introduction to the Practice of Clinical Hypnosis*. New York: Brunner/Mazel

Zahourek, R. (1990). *Clinical Hypnosis and Therapeutic Suggestion in Patient Care*. New York: Brunner/Mazel.

Zeig, J. K. (1980a). Symptom prescription and Ericksonian principles of hypnosis and psychotherapy. *American Journal of Clinical Hypnosis, 23*, 16–22.

Zeig, J. K. (1980b). Symptom prescription techniques: Clinical applications using elements of communication. *American Journal of Clinical Hypnosis, 23*, 23–33.

Zeig, J. K. (1980c). *A Teaching Seminar with Milton H. Erickson*. New York: Brunner/Mazel.

Index